The Natural Medicine Guide to

ADDICTION

Also by Stephanie Marohn

Natural Medicine First Aid Remedies

Other Titles in the **Healthy Mind Guide** Series:

The Natural Medicine Guide to Autism

The Natural Medicine Guide to Depression

The Natural Medicine Guide to Bipolar Disorder

The Natural Medicine Guide to Anxiety

The Natural Medicine Guide to Schizophrenia

THE HEALTHY ● MIND GUIDES

The Natural Medicine Guide to
ADDICTION

Stephanie Marohn

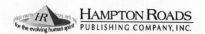

HAMPTON ROADS
PUBLISHING COMPANY, INC.

Cover design by Bookwrights Design
Cover art/photographic image © 2003 Loyd Chapplow
Interior MediClip images © Williams & Wilkins. All rights reserved.
Acupressure meridian and chakra illustrations
© 2004 Anne L. Louque. All rights reserved.

Hampton Roads Publishing Company, Inc.
1125 Stoney Ridge Road
Charlottesville, VA 22902

434-296-2772
fax: 434-296-5096
e-mail: hrpc@hrpub.com
www.hrpub.com

If you are unable to order this book from your local
bookseller, you may order directly from the publisher.
Call 1-800-766-8009, toll-free.

Library of Congress Cataloging-in-Publication Data

Marohn, Stephanie.
  The natural medicine guide to addiction / Stephanie Marohn.
     p. cm.
  Includes bibliographical references and index.
  ISBN 1-57174-290-5 (5 x 8 tp : alk. paper)
  1. Compulsive behavior--Alternative treatment. 2. Substance
abuse--Alternative treatment. I. Title.
  RC533.M37 2004
  616.86'06--dc22
                                    2004000742

ISBN 1-57174-290-5
10 9 8 7 6 5 4 3 2 1
Printed on acid-free paper in the United States

THE HEALTHY ● MIND GUIDES

The Healthy Mind Guides are a series of books offering original research and treatment options for reversing or ameliorating so-called mental disorders, written by noted health journalist and author Stephanie Marohn. The series' focus is the natural medicine approach, a refreshing and hopeful outlook based on treating individual needs rather than medical labels, and addressing the underlying imbalances—biological, psychological, emotional, and spiritual.

Each book in the series offers the very latest information about the possible causes of each disorder, and presents a wide range of effective, practical therapies drawn from extensive interviews with physicians and other practitioners who are innovators in their respective fields. Case studies throughout the books illustrate the applications of these therapies, and numerous resources are provided for readers who want to seek treatment.

༈

To my grandparents

Rachel Ziegler Green and Charles R. Green

Acknowledgments

My deep gratitude to all of the following:

The doctors and other healing professionals who shared information on their work for this book:

Ira J. Golchehreh, L.Ac., O.M.D.
William M. Hitt, Ph.D.
Patricia Kaminski
Dietrich Klinghardt, M.D., Ph.D.
Reverend Leon S. LeGant
Devi S. Nambudripad, M.D., D.C., L.Ac., Ph.D.
Tony Roffers, Ph.D.
Julia Ross, M.A.

Rhys and Mary Marohn for taking such good care of a writer on leave.

Mary Ford-Grabowsky and Dorothy Walters for company par excellence and life-path inspiration.

The Gaia Circle and my animal companions for seeing me spiritually through the writing of six books.

Donna Canali, Mella Mincberg, and Moli Steinert for life together.

Editor and friend Richard Leviton, as always.

The entire staff at Hampton Roads for putting the *Healthy Mind Guides* into the hands of those who need them.

Contents

Introduction

Substance abuse is a worldwide epidemic. In the United States alone, a 1993 survey found that heavy drinking was taking place in over 40 million households, illegal drug use in 14.5 million households, and abuse of prescription drugs in 3.5 million households.[1] Tobacco use around the world has increased by almost 75 percent in the past few decades.[2]

Substance abuse has become the number one health problem and the leading cause of death in the United States.[3] More than 100,000 deaths annually are related to alcohol. One in six deaths are caused by cigarette smoking. Every year 400,000 people die as a result of their cigarette smoking, while another 50,000 people die as a result of secondary smoke.[4] An estimated one-third of all hospital admissions, 25 percent of all deaths, and the majority of serious crimes are linked to drug, alcohol, or cigarette addiction.[5] One-third of all suicides, more than 50 percent of homicides and domestic violence incidents, and 25 percent of emergency room admissions are related to alcohol.[6]

These statistics reflect the dire consequences and high cost of substance addictions only. There are millions more people around the world who suffer from behavioral or activity addictions that are resulting in serious physical, psychological, occupational, financial, interpersonal, and other consequences in their lives. Among these addictions are compulsive eating, gambling, sexual activity, working, exercising, spending, and Internet use—the emphasis being on compulsive.

The "war" on drugs has done nothing to end the epidemic of substance abuse. It has only resulted in filling prisons. The prison population in the United States mushroomed from 500,000 in 1980 to over two million in 2000.[7]

For the most part, those imprisoned do not receive treatment for problems with substance abuse. While 43 percent of new arrestees in U.S. city jails reported an alcohol or drug abuse problem needing treatment (the percentage is likely far higher as it does not reflect those who did not admit to having a problem), only 28 percent of the jails offer such treatment, mainly AA meetings. In state prisons, two-thirds of prisoners needing drug treatment are not getting it, with only about 11 percent enrolled in programs.[8]

Substance abuse, inside and outside prisons, continues unabated.

Addiction is part of a triumvirate of mental health epidemics currently afflicting the world, with anxiety and depression being the other two. The incidence of anxiety disorders rose dramatically in the second half of the twentieth century, to the point that they are now the most common "mental" illness.[9]

In a given year, one in nine Americans are now suffering from an anxiety disorder.[10] Depression is rising at an equally alarming rate. In the United States alone, 30 million people are taking Prozac, which is now in the top ten most prescribed drugs.[11] That translates to nearly one in ten people. A study by the World Health Organization (WHO) and the Harvard School of Public Health reveals that by the year 2020 depression will be the single leading cause of death around the globe.[12]

The dramatic rise in addiction, anxiety, and depression around the globe is not a parallel occurrence. These are not separate epidemics, but intertwined disorders. As you will learn in this book, anxiety and depression are the unaddressed, underlying disorders of addiction. The failure to treat these disorders helps explain the abysmal statistics of conventional addiction treatment: 50 to 90 percent of alcoholics and drug addicts relapse (the percentage varies with the statistical source); and almost 25 percent of the deaths among people treated for chemical dependency are suicides.[13]

Depression and anxiety have both been clearly linked to suicide.

As valuable a contribution as Twelve-Step programs (Alcoholics Anonymous and others) make in providing peer support and a structure for addiction recovery, a research review of comparative studies

Introduction

of standard treatment approaches, including AA, revealed that there is "little or no evidence of effectiveness."[14] Two studies in the review showed that alcoholics "did no better or actually suffered more relapse" with AA than those who got other or no treatment.[15] This is not to undercut the importance of Twelve-Step programs in addiction recovery, but to point out that something is missing from our current addiction treatment model.

The Natural Medicine Guide to Addiction explores what is missing in that model. Although addiction is now viewed as a physiological brain disorder, amazingly, conventional treatment does not address the physical aspect of the problem. While addiction is compared to diabetes to legitimize its status as a disease, no physical treatment is forthcoming. Antidepressant and antianxiety drugs are touted for relief from mood disturbances and psychotherapy and/or Twelve-Step groups for support in maintaining sobriety. Where is the treatment?

This book fills the gap of this gigantic omission by exploring a range of natural therapies that address the physical as well as the psychological and spiritual aspects of addiction. Deficiencies in the nutrients that feed vital brain

The book offers a range of treatment approaches to address these factors and truly restore health. Only by considering the well-being of the body, mind, and spirit can comprehensive healing take place, which is evidenced by the far higher success rate of this model (as high as 95 percent in the case of the work of Dr. William M. Hitt; see chapter 3).

chemicals, other nutritional deficiencies, allergies, hypoglycemia (low blood sugar), and toxicity are among the physical factors considered. These factors can be operational in all types of addiction: alcoholism, addiction to street or prescription drugs, and eating and other behavioral addictions.

The book covers the gamut of types of addiction and is dedicated to exploring the underlying causal and contributing factors, with the goal of healing from addiction, rather than accepting the lifetime label of "alcoholic" or "addict." To this end, the book offers a range of treatment approaches to address these factors and truly restore health. Only by considering the well-being of the body, mind, and spirit can comprehensive healing take place, which is evidenced by the far higher success rate of this model (as high as 95 percent in the case of the work of Dr. William M. Hitt; see chapter 3).

All of the therapies covered here approach the treatment of addiction in this way. They all also share the characteristic of tailoring treatment to the individual, which is another essential element for a successful outcome. No two people, even with the same addiction, have exactly the same imbalances causing their problems.

With the increase in the number of people who are using natural therapies, the public has become more aware of this medical approach. When many people think of natural medicine, however, they think of supplements or herbal remedies available over the counter. While these products can be highly beneficial, natural medicine is far more than that. Natural therapies are those that operate according to holistic principles, meaning treating the whole person rather than an isolated part or symptom and using natural treatments that "Do no harm" and support or restore the body's natural ability to heal itself.

Natural medicine involves a way of looking at healing that is dramatically different from the conventional medical model. It does not mimic that model by merely substituting the herbal medicine kava-kava for an antianxiety drug or St. John's wort for an antidepressant drug. Instead, it is the comprehensive approach described above, which offers you the very real possibility of curing your addiction.

Herbal and other natural remedies can be a useful corollary in alleviating the anxiety and depression associated with addiction, however. As there is already ample information on natural remedies for anxiety and depression and it doesn't fit with the in-depth treatment focus of this book, I don't cover such remedies here. (For self-help treatments for anxiety and depression, see my book *Natural Medicine First Aid Remedies,* Hampton Roads, 2001.)

Before I tell you a little about what's in the book, I would just like to say a few words about the terms "mental illness" and "mental disorders," or "brain disorders" as they are more currently labeled. All of these terms reflect the disconnection between body and mind—never mind spirit—in conventional medical treatment. The newer term, brain disorders, reflects the biochemical model of causality that currently dominates the medical profession.

I use the terms "mental disorders" and "brain disorders" in this book because there is no easy substitute that reflects the true body-mind-spirit nature of these conditions. While I may use these terms, I in no way mean to suggest that the causes of the disorders lie solely in the mind or brain. The same is true for the title of the series of which this book is a part: the *Healthy Mind Guides*. The name serves to distinguish the subject area, but it is healthy mind, body, and spirit—wholeness—that is the focus of these books.

While I'm at it, I may as well dispense with one last linguistic issue. As natural medicine effects profound healing, rather than simply controlling symptoms, I prefer the term "natural medicine" over "alternative medicine." This medical model is not "other"—it is a primary form of medicine. The term "holistic medicine" reflects this as well, in that it signals the natural medicine approach of treating the whole person, rather than the parts.

Part 1 of *The Natural Medicine Guide to Addiction* covers the basics of addiction: what it is, who suffers from it, and what causes or contributes to it. The natural medicine view is that many different factors (physical, psychological, and spiritual), often in combination, contribute to addiction.

Part 2 of the book covers a range of natural medicine treatments for addiction. The material presented here is based on research and interviews with physicians and other healing professionals who are leaders and pioneers in their respective fields. This is original information, not derivative material gleaned from secondary sources. The therapeutic techniques of these highly skilled doctors and other healers are explained in detail and illustrated with case studies that give a human face to addiction and demonstrate the effectiveness of the therapies. (The names of patients throughout the book have been changed. Contact information for the practitioners whose work is presented appears in the resource appendix.)

The types of addiction featured in cases throughout the book include addiction to alcohol, prescription drugs, street drugs (cocaine, crack, crystal meth, marijuana, and ecstasy), tobacco, sex, and food. Here is a sample of the successful recoveries that are possible with the natural medicine approach to addiction:

- After a ten-day intensive biochemical treatment, Celeste, 38, was able to end her serious, long-term crystal meth habit that had resisted all other treatment approaches.

- Susan, 56, overcame her out-of-control drinking with acupuncture treatments and a Chinese herbal medicine protocol; her cravings for alcohol were gone after two acupuncture sessions.

- Flower essence therapy helped Jeremy, 29, leave his marijuana addiction behind and get on with his life.

- Estelle, in her fifties, quit her lifetime pack-a-day smoking habit after three treatments to clear her allergies, notably to tobacco, vitamin B-complex, and sugar.

- Mike, in his early forties, had no more problems with smoking and sex addiction after he cleared the allergies and uncovered the trauma behind them through advanced energy-based psychotherapeutic techniques.

Part 2 begins with chapter 3 and an exploration of one of the most striking physical treatments for addiction, which scientists have known about for decades but which conventional treatment has chosen to ignore. It is amino acid therapy, delivered as simple oral supplements or in intravenous formulas. Amino acids are the building blocks of protein and vital for proper brain chemistry. This therapy addresses the biological brain disorder that science views as the cause of addiction.

Chapter 4 explores the role of allergies in addiction, another physical factor that is almost entirely overlooked in addiction treatment. Chapters 5 and 6 look at two different kinds of energy-based medicine: traditional Chinese medicine and flower essence therapy. Unlike drugs or nutritional supplements, which operate on a biochemical or physical level, these therapies function on an energetic level to reverse the energy imbalances contributing to addiction and restore the equilibrium of the body, mind, and spirit. Energy medicine is little understood in the West, and these chapters present the power of this form of medicine in clear and accessible language.

Chapter 7 presents a model of healing that delineates the five levels of a person that must be restored to balance if complete health and well-being are to be achieved. The five levels—Physical, Electromagnetic, Mental, Intuitive, and Spiritual—are explored in depth, along with how problems at different levels can produce addiction and the therapies that can be used to reverse them.

Among the featured therapies in this chapter is Family Systems Therapy, an innovative technique to address transgenerational issues that is widely practiced in Europe and just beginning to become known in the United States. This chapter provides a framework for approaching recovery from addiction as well as for understanding how the natural medicine therapies described in the other chapters work to address the whole person.

Chapter 8 explores the role of trauma and anxiety in addiction. It details how two energy-based psychotherapies—Thought Field Therapy and Seemorg Matrix Work—can resolve trauma from the past far more quickly than standard psychotherapeutic methods. These leading-edge therapies, which came onto the psychotherapeutic scene in the 1990s, were both developed by psychotherapists who were frustrated by the lack of results in standard practice.

The last chapter in part 2 focuses on psychospiritual contributions to addiction and turns to psychic healing for its insightful analysis of the disorder. Psychic healing, also known as spiritual healing, considers the role of foreign energies in preventing spiritual connection and creating addiction, and works to clear them.

The combination of therapies found in these chapters and covering the spectrum of body, mind, and spirit factors in addiction is unique. By offering a comprehensive and deep approach to healing, these therapies have the potential to help you find your way to an addiction-free life.

Natural Medicine Therapies Covered in Part II

Chap.	Health Practitioner	Therapies
3	Julia Ross, M.A. Dr. William M. Hitt	Amino acid therapy Neurotransmitter Restoration
4	Devi S. Nambudripad, M.D., D.C., L.Ac., Ph.D.	NAET (allergy testing and elimination; includes MRT, muscle response testing)
5	Ira J. Golchehreh, L.Ac., O.M.D.	Traditional Chinese medicine Acupuncture Herbal medicine
6	Patricia Kaminski	Flower essence therapy
7	Dietrich Klinghardt, M.D., Ph.D.	APN (Applied Psychoneuro- biology) Chelation/heavy metal detoxification Family Systems Therapy NAET (allergy elimination) Thought Field Therapy
8	Tony Roffers, Ph.D.	Seemorg Matrix Work Thought Field Therapy
9	Rev. Leon S. LeGant	Spiritual/psychic healing

PART I

The Basics of Addiction

1 What Is Addiction and Who Suffers from It?

"Addiction is a physical disease."[16]

"Addiction is a misguided search for self-love and spiritual fulfillment."[17]

"We can draw a strong comparison between addiction and cancer."[18]

"Addiction is an active belief in and a commitment to a negative lifestyle."[19]

"Addiction is a disease which, without recovery, ends in jails, institutions, and death."[20]

"Addiction is a continuum; your behavior is more or less addicted."[21]

"In its beginning stages, addiction is an attempt to emotionally fulfill oneself."[22]

"Addiction is a disorder of the brain no different from other forms of mental illness."[23]

"Chemical dependency . . . is a chronic disease that has no cure."[24]

As you can see from the above definitions of addiction, all offered by professionals in the field of addiction treatment today, there is a wide range of opinion on what exactly addiction is. Conventional psychiatry and Twelve-Step programs subscribe to the incurable disease model, which holds that "Once an addict, always an addict." The natural medicine approach regards addiction as the consequence of physical, energetic, psychological, and/or spiritual imbalances that can be corrected. Everyone agrees, however, that untreated addiction affects every aspect of life and has far-reaching consequences. It also cuts across all class, race, and gender lines. Addiction is an equal opportunity affliction.

The complexity and scope of the problem of addiction are reflected in the fact that the *DSM-IV (Diagnostic and Statistical Manual of Mental Disorders, 4th Edition),* the American Psychiatric Association's diagnostic bible for psychiatric disorders, devotes over 100 pages to "substance-related disorders" alone, more than is allocated to any of the other so-called mental disorders covered in the text.

Amidst these 100 pages, substance dependence (the clinical term for substance addiction) is defined broadly as "a cluster of cognitive, behavioral, and physiological symptoms indicating that the individual continues use of the substance despite significant substance-related problems."[25] More specifically, to meet the criteria for a diagnosis of substance dependence, at least three of the following must be operational in the space of a year:[26]

- Tolerance (either a need for more of the substance or reduced effects from the same amount)

- Withdrawal when discontinuing use of the substance, or taking the substance (or one like it) to avoid or relieve withdrawal symptoms

- Taking more of the substance or for longer than intended

- Desire or failed attempts to reduce or control substance use

- Much time dedicated to obtaining, using, or recovering from use of the substance

- Giving up or reducing social, professional, or leisure activities due to substance use

- Continuing to use substance despite physical or psychological problems related to its use

In other words, the person experiences a loss of control and has a compulsion to use despite adverse consequences. The *DSM-IV* distinguishes between substance dependence and substance abuse. For a diagnosis of substance abuse, at least one of the following must be present in the space of a year:[27]

- Failure to meet professional or familial obligations as a result of recurrent substance use

- Recurrent substance use in situations in which it is physically dangerous to use, as when driving or operating machinery

- Recurrent legal problems related to substance use

- Continuing to use substance despite social or interpersonal problems related to its use

The main difference between substance dependence and abuse, then, according to these definitions, is the physiological component of addiction, as manifested in the points regarding tolerance, withdrawal, loss of control, and the nature of the adverse results. This difference may simply be one of

Addicted America

- Approximately 18 million Americans have alcohol problems and 5 to 6 million have drug problems.[28]

- 53 percent of American adults have a family history of alcoholism or problem drinking.[29]

- 14.8 million Americans use illegal drugs[30]

- 1 to 2 million are regular methamphetamine (speed) users[31]

- Among Americans over 12 years old, 5 percent report using marijuana every month, and 1.8 percent use cocaine monthly.[32]

- The annual cost of substance abuse in the United States is an estimated $276 billion (which includes the cost of healthcare, lost productivity, crime, and motor vehicle accidents).[33]

- Untreated addiction costs more than heart disease, diabetes, and cancer combined.[34]

- The damages from addiction cost every American adult almost $1,000 per year.[35]

degree or stages of substance use, or it may be due to the presence or absence of factors that predispose an individual to develop full-blown addiction (see chapter 2). In any case, the line between abuse and dependence is not always clear and need not be to initiate treatment. Many addiction-treatment providers do not make the distinction. The therapeutic approaches discussed in this book have equal application to abuse or dependence (and to substances and behaviors).

While the *DSM-IV* covers only problems with substances, aside from pathological gambling, which is discussed under "Impulse-Control Disorders," many of those in the addiction treatment field categorize addiction as two types: substance addictions and process addictions. The former includes addictions to alcohol, tobacco, and illegal and prescription drugs, while the latter covers behavioral or activity addictions, such as eating, gambling, spending, working, exercising, and sexual activity addictions.

While people may start using a substance or activity to feel good, addiction progresses to the point that they *must* use to keep from feeling bad. "Addicts become addicted not because of the high, but because they need their substance to satisfy their physiological hunger, to relieve the symptoms of depression, and to stave off withdrawal symptoms," states Janice Keller Phelps, M.D., a specialist in the treatment of addiction since 1977.[36]

Withdrawal symptoms vary according to the nature of the addiction, from mood disturbances such as anxiety, depression, agitation, mood swings, irritability, and restlessness to physical symptoms such as chills, shaking, profuse sweating, and abdominal pain. Withdrawal is not necessarily over after conventional detoxification is complete. Post-acute withdrawal syndrome (PAWS), which can include the mood disturbances above as well as insomnia, listlessness, malaise, and/or headaches, can occur as long as a year and a half after "detoxification."[37]

The term "detoxification" as it is employed conventionally does not entail an active detoxification protocol, but simply refers to the process of detoxification or withdrawal that the body does on its own when the formerly abused substance is withheld.

In part 2, you will learn about the biochemistry of withdrawal and how the nightmare of symptoms associated with it can be avoided with amino acids and other nutrients, among other natural medicine therapies. Rebalancing the biochemistry makes it possible for the individual to have the mental and physical wherewithal to proceed to

Addiction Categories

Substance Addictions

- Stimulants (uppers): amphetamines (amphetamine, methamphetamine, dextroamphetamine), methylphenidate (Ritalin), cocaine, crack, caffeine, alcohol, nicotine*

- Depressants (downers): sedatives (barbiturates), hypnotics, benzodiazepines (tranquilizers, sleeping pills), anxiolytics (anti-anxiety drugs), alcohol, nicotine

- Opioids: heroin, opium, morphine, and prescription narcotic painkillers such as codeine, Dilaudid, Darvon, Demerol, Percodan, and Vicodin

- Other drugs: cannabinoids (marijuana, hashish), PCP (angel dust), hallucinogens (LSD, mescaline, psilocybin mushrooms), steroids

- Inhalants: paint thinner, glue, gasoline, nitrous oxide (laughing gas), propane, poppers

Process Addictions

- Eating (food addiction), sexual activity (sex addiction), relationships, workaholism, exercise, gambling, compulsive spending, Internet addiction

*Note that alcohol and nicotine are both stimulants and depressants.

addressing the behavioral, emotional, and spiritual aspects of their addiction as well. A lack of understanding of the multifaceted nature of addiction is what typically makes addiction recovery difficult.

Types of Addiction

There are two main categories of addiction high: arousal and satiation. The arousal high is about temporarily feeling omnipotent. The satiation high is about numbing pain. Substances and activities that produce the arousal high include speed, cocaine, ecstasy (MDMA), Ritalin (used by adults), alcohol during the first few drinks, gambling, and sex addiction activities. Those that produce the satiation high include heroin, alcohol, marijuana, tranquilizers, and food addiction behaviors.[38]

Another way to describe the categories is: substances and behaviors that stimulate nervous system activity and substances and behaviors that depress nervous system activity. Substances can be further broken down into specific drug categories, such as stimulants, depressants, opioids, hallucinogens, cannabinoids, and steroids. Although different substances produce different problems in association with addiction, many practitioners believe that addiction is addiction and all "types" must be treated in the same basic way. Not acknowledging this fact promotes the substitution of one addiction for another. For example, using Valium (diazepam) to help people quit drinking often results in a Valium addiction.[39]

Information about the various categories of addiction and substance abuse is helpful in understanding addiction, however. Here we look at alcohol, street drugs, prescription drugs, tobacco, and common addictive behaviors/activities.

Alcohol

Abuse of alcohol is rampant: 18 million Americans have alcohol problems[40] and 53 percent of American adults have a family history of alcoholism or problem drinking.[41]

Alcoholism varies crossculturally, however. Research has found that Native Americans and the Irish have very high rates of alcoholism, while Chinese, Greeks, Italians, and Jews have very low rates. Some researchers suggest that this is due to differences in how the cultures view alcohol.

For example, the Irish tend to view drinking in all-or-nothing terms while Mediterranean cultures exhibit a more moderate attitude. In the latter, drinking takes place within the family and "doesn't carry the emotional baggage that drinking does for groups with a greater susceptibility to alcoholism," states Stanton Peele, Ph.D., a psychologist, researcher, and specialist in the field of addiction.[42]

In addiction treatment, the term alcoholism has come to refer to both alcohol abuse and dependence, a reflection of the fine line that separates them. The prevailing medical model holds that alcoholism is a physical disease that when untreated results in bio-psycho-social damage, meaning that the body, mind, and interpersonal relationships are affected. Social damage encompasses family, friends, career, and community.

Alcohol is slightly unusual in that it can act as both a stimulant and depressant. For the first few drinks, it is a stimulant; with further drinking, it becomes a depressant. As with drugs, alcohol produces its effects by acting on the brain's neurotransmitters (chemical messengers). Its pleasurable effects are likely the result of its action on endorphins, the body's natural painkillers and the source of "runner's high." Alcohol's sedative effects are likely due to its action on GABA (gamma-aminobutyric acid), which has a calming effect on the brain.

Another neurotransmitter involved is dopamine. Known as one of the "feel good" neurotransmitters, meaning that it is their presence and function that enable us to be in a good mood, its release in the brain is connected to the sensations of satisfaction and euphoria. Later in the chapter dopamine is discussed in more depth because research indicates that it is the primary neurotransmitter involved in all forms of addiction.

A further effect of alcohol on normal neurotransmitter function is that it impedes the supply of tryptophan (the amino acid precursor to the neurotransmitter serotonin) to the brain and thus reduces serotonin formation. Serotonin is involved in mood regulation, and disturbances in its levels or function have been linked to depression and anxiety, which offers an explanation for why these two mood states often coexist with alcohol abuse.

In addition to anxiety and depression, symptoms of alcohol abuse include facial puffiness, spider-like capillary formations on the face, flushing, sweating, dyspepsia, sleep problems, tremors, and chronic fatigue. The symptoms depend upon the severity of the drinking problem.

Withdrawal symptoms likewise depend upon the degree of abuse and can include increased heart rate, elevated blood pressure, anxiety, nausea, vomiting, headache, sweating, tremors, seizures, confusion, disorientation, hallucinations, and anxiety ranging from mild agitation in less severe cases to panic in more severe cases. The most severe withdrawal is termed "delirium tremens," or DTs.

The consequences of alcohol abuse are far-reaching. It can potentially damage every system of the body. Organ damage, cirrhosis of the liver, high blood pressure, heart problems, nutritional deficiencies, gastrointestinal problems (ulcers and gastritis), immune suppression,

Is Your Substance Use a Problem?

The CAGE test is an informal method for determining whether substance abuse may be a problem for you. Answer the following four questions:

Have you ever tried to **C**ut down on your drinking (drug use)?

Have you ever felt **A**nnoyed by someone's comments about your drinking (drug use)?

Have you ever felt **G**uilty or concerned about your drinking (drug use)?

Have you ever had an **E**ye-opener drink (or a drug to avoid or ease withdrawal symptoms) in the morning?

(The questions can be modified slightly to apply to process addictions, as in: Have you ever tried to cut down on your gambling/ shopping/Internet use?)

Some practitioners say that a "yes" answer to one or more of the questions may indicate a possible problem; others say that "yes" to two or more suggests dependence. The test is obviously far from definitive but can serve as a starting point for considering the issue of addiction.

hormonal dysfunction, neurological damage, organic brain syndrome (permanent memory impairment), and possibly increased risk of certain types of cancer can all result from excess drinking.[43]

Alcoholism is the third leading cause of death in the United States.[44] More than 100,000 deaths annually are related to alcohol.[45] One-third of all suicides, over 50 percent of homicides and domestic violence incidents, and 25 percent of emergency room admissions are related to alcohol.[46]

The recovery rate with conventional treatment of alcoholism is low, ranging from 15 to 30 percent, depending on the source. The relapse rate among alcoholics is high, with half of those who go through treatment relapsing at least once.[47]

Street Drugs

Like alcohol, the use of illegal drugs is woven into the fabric of American society. An estimated 14.8 million Americans use illegal drugs[48] and five to six million Americans have drug problems.[49] One to two million use methamphetamine (speed) regularly[50] and 1.8 percent of Americans over the age of 12 use cocaine monthly.[51] Five percent of those over 12 years old report using marijuana every month.[52] Eight percent of high school seniors report that they have tried ecstasy (MDMA, methylenedioxymethamphetamine) at least once.[53] Nearly 80 percent of Americans have tried illegal drugs by the time they are in their mid-twenties.[54]

The stimulant drugs speed (amphetamine, methamphetamine, and dextroamphetamine), cocaine, and crack; the opioids heroin, opium, and morphine; the cannabinoids marijuana and hashish; the hallucinogens LSD, mescaline, and psilocybin mushrooms; and phencyclidine (PCP, angel dust) can all be the source of substance abuse. While not technically drugs, substances inhaled for intoxification purposes include paint thinner, glue, gasoline, nitrous oxide (laughing gas), propane gas, and amyl and butyl nitrate (poppers).

As with alcohol, all of these drugs are thought to affect the dopamine neurotransmitter system, among other neurotransmitters. Speed, for example, floods the brain with dopamine, and scientists have found that even low levels of methamphetamine over time can damage up to 50 percent of the dopamine-producing cells in the brain.[55] One study found that the level of dopamine in methamphetamine addicts was 24 percent lower than in normal subjects.[56]

Heroin and marijuana also trigger dopamine release. Cocaine and crack block the absorption of dopamine, resulting in more dopamine in circulation in the brain. Chronic use damages dopamine receptors and disturbs the regulation of pleasure. (Receptors are the components of nerve cells that receive the neurotransmitter.)

While amphetamines are prescription drugs, illicit speed is used in a variety of ways, from shooting up to smoking it, which takes it out of the realm of "popping a pill." Street speed is also so prevalent that it must be included here as a street drug. Methamphetamine (known as crystal meth or crystal) use is on the rise around the world. In Thailand, for example, it is the "working man's and woman's preferred intoxicant," and according to an investigating writer for *Time* magazine, in one Bangkok slum of 5,000 residents it is difficult on weekends to find anyone who is not high on *yaba* (mad medicine), the local name for meth.[57]

Speed is neurotoxic, meaning toxic to the nervous system, and chronic use can produce rapid or irregular heartbeat, weight loss, malnutrition, insomnia, irritability, restlessness, anxiety, panic, paranoia, psychosis, loss of coordination, tremors, seizures, stroke, and heart failure.

Heroin and other opiates operate on the brain's natural painkillers, endorphins and enkephalins. With heroin use, the body makes less of these substances and tries to reduce the effects of the introduced opiates. The result is higher doses of heroin are needed to produce a high. The primary health consequences of heroin abuse, in addition to the risk of overdose and the contraction of HIV from sharing needles, are respiratory depression and arrest, confusion, insomnia, anxiety, and depression.

Although much has been made of the horrors of heroin withdrawal, addicts report that a severe illness such as hepatitis B is much worse.[58]

Many also report that it is more difficult to give up cigarettes. The focus on heroin as the bogeyman of withdrawal overshadows the real dangers of withdrawal from Valium and other benzodiazepines, which unlike heroin can be life-threatening. With any drug, if the natural medicine therapies you will learn about in part 2 were instituted in detoxification centers everywhere, withdrawal as we have known it would be a thing of the past.

While marijuana is regarded by many as a harmless drug, 10 to 15 percent of marijuana users become dependent on it, that is, are unable to give it up.[59] In the brain, marijuana binds to receptor sites in areas that regulate mood and memory. Impaired memory and learning, anxiety, and panic attacks are among the health consequences of chronic marijuana use. Other consequences include frequent respiratory infections, cough, and elevated heart rate.[60]

Cocaine is generally considered today to be one of the most addictive drugs there are, and as a result nearly impossible for addicts to quit on their own.[61]

There is research contradicting this view, however, and critics of this widely disseminated position point out that the same used to be said of heroin, which has since proven false. In reality, no illicit drug is inherently addictive, as evidenced by studies demonstrating that not everyone who uses these drugs becomes addicted and the majority of those who use drugs on a regular basis do not become addicted.[62]

This evidence underscores the fact that in order to identify the causes of addiction one must *look to the individual* rather than to the drug. Chapter 2 explores the multiple factors that can contribute to the development of addiction.

As with other substance abuse, cocaine addiction can have serious health consequences, including chest pain, respiratory failure, nausea, abdominal pain, headaches, insomnia, weight loss, malnutrition, anxiety, panic, paranoia, psychosis, tremors, seizures, stroke, and heart failure.

Cocaine, amphetamines, PCP, hallucinogens, and inhalants are sources of substance-induced anxiety disorders and can worsen already existing anxiety.[63] Habitual use of cocaine and amphetamines, for example, can interfere with production of the neurotransmitters that inhibit irritability and other heightened reactivity, leading to excessive anxiety.[64] Narcotics, which people may use in an attempt to self-medicate anxiety, can actually worsen it.[65] People with panic disorder frequently cite the use of marijuana as the "single initiatory factor" in the first attack they experienced.[66]

Prescription Drugs

In addition to iatrogenic (physician-induced) addictions, which means that a doctor prescribed the drug to which you are addicted, prescription drug abuse occurs through illegal channels as well. The following are categories of drugs that are commonly abused, whether they are obtained through legal or illegal means: amphetamines, sedatives (barbiturates), hypnotics, benzodiazepines (tranquilizers, sleeping pills), anxiolytics (anti-anxiety drugs), steroids, and the narcotic analgesics (painkillers such as codeine, Dilaudid, Darvon, Demerol, Percodan, and Vicodin).

The prevalence in abuse of prescription drugs is reflected in the cultural milieu. One joke making the rounds refers to the ubiquitous use of Xanax (alprazolam), pronounced *zanax*, an anti-anxiety drug: The drink of choice these days is the Zanatini, a martini with a Xanax-stuffed olive.[67] The painkiller Vicodin has become the trendy drug that cocaine was in the 1990s. The subject of pop songs and featured as a tattoo on the arm of platinum-selling rapper Eminem, Vicodin has become "the narcotic of choice for the celebrity set."[68]

The illicit use of painkillers in general has risen dramatically throughout the United States. The number of Americans who began taking prescription painkillers for "nonmedical" purposes nearly tripled from 1990 to 1998 to a record 1.5 million, as reported by the Department of Health and Human Services.[69]

The greatest risk factor for abuse of prescription drugs is an existing alcohol or drug problem.[70] Those in recovery are also at risk. Richard Rogg, founder and owner of Promises Malibu, a rehab facility near Los Angeles that caters to celebrity clients, states, "I'm hearing the same old story: 'I had five or ten years' sobriety, but I got loaded on Vicodin, and I went out.'"[71]

The prevalence in abuse of prescription drugs is reflected in the cultural milieu. One joke making the rounds refers to the ubiquitous use of Xanax (alprazolam), pronounced zanax, an anti-anxiety drug: The drink of choice these days is the Zanatini, a martini with a Xanax-stuffed olive.

Nonmedical use of Rohypnol (flunitrazepam) is also on the rise. It is a sleeping pill in the same class of drugs as Valium and Xanax (benzodiazepines) but is ten times more powerful than Valium. Though Rohypnol is illegal in the United States, it is sold by prescription in over 60 other countries and so is available as a street drug in the U.S.[72] One of its street names is *papas,* Spanish for "potatoes," a reflection of the user's mental capacity while on the drug.[73] Anxiety, insomnia, tremor, elevated blood pressure, seizures, and increased sensitivity to light, touch, and sound are among the withdrawal symptoms.[74]

Ritalin (methylphenidate), the amphetamine that record numbers of children are being given for ADHD (attention deficit/hyperactivity disorder), is an increasing source of adult drug abuse. In adults, it acts on the brain in a manner similar to cocaine. "Having practiced addiction medicine for many years, let me relay to you what my stimulant-addicted patients have to say about Ritalin," says Charles Gant, M.D., Ph.D., of East Syracuse, New York. "They call it the "cognac of speed," the "best stuff," and the "nicest high of all the uppers."[75]

Ritalin has also been dubbed the "poor man's cocaine" and is used by college students pulling "all-nighters."[76] Some of the indicators of abuse are depression, anxiety, insomnia, chronic pain, and headaches.[77]

> ## In Their Own Words
>
> *"After two years I am finally back in working order. I am finally able to concentrate without Ritalin. But suffice it to say my life at age 32 in no way resembles the one I had pictured before addiction became a part of it. And all this as a result of this little pill that is safe enough to give to preschoolers. Imagine that."*
>
> —Elizabeth Wurtzel, on her Ritalin addiction[79]

Author Elizabeth Wurtzel, who wrote about her experiences with a Ritalin addiction in an article in the *New York Times,* reports that she was given a Ritalin prescription to enhance the action of her anti-depressant medication. She was soon addicted and taking high doses every day. She ended up spending four months in a residential treatment center followed by six months of participation in an outpatient program in order to get off the drug. In Narcotics Anonymous meetings, other Ritalin addicts included those who had been prescribed the drug as a child and mothers who would steal pills from their children's prescription.[78]

Tobacco

Like drugs and alcohol, nicotine (in cigarettes, snuff, and chewing tobacco) affects neurotransmitters. Research suggests that nicotine has similar effects on the brain to cocaine.[80] Specifically, it triggers dopamine release and blocks the action of the enzyme that breaks down dopamine, resulting in a greater circulation of the "feel good" neurotransmitter. Like alcohol, it acts as both a stimulant and depressant, which explains the role of smoking as both a calming and pleasure-producing activity.

This may explain why it is so difficult to quit smoking, along with the fact that as most smokers started in their teens, the habit tends to be ingrained and smoking is integrated into so many activities of daily life. Addicts have rated it the hardest drug to give up.[81] Nevertheless, over 40 million former smokers no longer do so, and 90 percent of those who quit manage to accomplish it on their own.[82]

Despite the fact that the health consequences of smoking are well documented, more than 50 million Americans still smoke. Over 50,000 studies have linked smoking to lung cancer, emphysema, heart disease, and pregnancy complications.[83] One in six deaths are caused by cigarette smoking. Every year 400,000 people die as a result of their cigarette smoking, while another 50,000 people die as a result of secondary smoke.[84]

Common Addictive Behaviors/Activities

Among the common behavior and activity addictions are food addiction, sex addiction (compulsive sexual activity), compulsive spending, compulsive Internet use, workaholism, addiction to relationships, exercise addiction, and gambling addiction.

The continuum of addiction is especially applicable to this category of addiction. It could be maintained that we all have addictions to some degree. Escaping through watching television, eating chocolate, or surfing the Internet are what some term "soft addictions," simply milder forms of self-medication than alcohol or drug addiction.[85] When such activities result in negative physical, mental, interpersonal, professional, or social consequences, they move out of the realm of soft addictions.

Based on the prevalence of obesity in the United States, Dr. Stanton Peele observes that "the substance problem that seems to be the most out of control for Americans is food."[86]

Research has shown that a high consumption of fat and sugar can disturb brain chemistry and cause addictive cravings for these substances.[87]

As you will learn later in this book, there is a body of evidence supporting the idea that sugar addiction sets the stage for all other addictions. Sugar is a simple carbohydrate, and it is thought that the addiction is caused by dysfunction in carbohydrate metabolism. Alcohol is also a simple carbohydrate. This model may explain the tremendous sugar cravings experienced by alcoholics and other addicts when they go off their substance of choice.

Sex addiction is also quite common and can take a number of forms. Compulsively engaging in sex, masturbation, sadomasochistic activity, pornography viewing, and sexual fantasies or obsessions are all aspects of sex addiction.

Compulsive reading of romance novels could be placed in this category as well. While it may seem innocuous on the surface, it can be a destructive addiction. As one woman who also struggles with compulsive sexual activity explains it: "The underlying message in romance novels is that there is a perfect someone out there for you and you find it through an encounter of immediate attraction that results in incredible, mind-blowing sex. I have found myself reading the same novels over and over again, but when I do this, I'm looking only for the sexual encounters. I keep the books with the most titillating scenes readily accessible. These scenes leave me either more tense and unsatisfied or masturbating. The end result is not at all fulfilling, and I feel like a kid sneaking a peak at dirty magazines. I know that since I've been reading romance novels I look at men in an even more conflicted way than before. I feel further away from reality than ever before."[88]

Another form of addictive escape is a phenomenon of the technological age. Internet addiction, or "chronic cyberphilia," has become such a problem that Internet addiction centers and specialists are now treating it.[89]

Maressa Hecht Orzack, Ph.D., a clinical psychologist at Harvard Medical School who works with computer addiction, states that the addiction coexists with at least one other disorder in all of her patients. "Depression, social phobia, impulse control disorder, and attention deficit disorder are commonest," she says.

Other addictions are also common. Research has found that Internet addicts are more likely than non-addicts to drink alcohol or use amphetamines, and pornography access may be a factor for a significant number of Internet addicts.[90] The addiction can progress to the point of loss of control, as with any other addiction. "Internet addicts can lose their jobs as they become unable to limit their time spent online, either because they fail to turn up for work or because they misuse their office computer facilities," says Dr. Orzack.

Multiple Addictions and Comorbidity

Multiple addictions, known clinically as polysubstance dependence, are common among addicts. Among alcoholics and drug abusers, independent research studies have found that 80 to 90 percent smoke cigarettes.[91] As noted earlier, an existing alcohol or drug problem is the greatest risk factor for abuse of prescription drugs. The incidence of sex addiction is higher among substance abusers than among the general population.[92]

There is an "extremely high" comorbidity between substance abuse and trauma.[93] Comorbidity means that two or more disorders exist together. One study of drug-abusing teenagers revealed that 77 percent of the girls and 45 percent of the boys had been sexually abused.[94] Other research demonstrated that childhood sexual abuse was far more common among women alcoholics than women who did not have a drinking problem.[95]

Similarly, there is a high comorbidity between addiction and mental disorders. ADD (attention deficit disorder) and addiction show a strong linkage. The risk of adult substance abuse is four to five times greater among children with untreated ADD than among non-ADD children.[96] As addiction is a form of obsession-compulsion, symptoms of obsessive-compulsive disorder (OCD) can emerge in early recovery.[97] OCD is characterized by persistent thoughts (obsessions) and repetitive or ritualistic behaviors or mental acts (compulsions).

As discussed earlier, addicts are often afflicted with depression and anxiety. The reverse is true as well. Among people who suffer from anxiety disorders, substance abuse is common; these disorders include panic disorder, social anxiety disorder (social phobia), specific (simple) phobia, generalized anxiety disorder (GAD), and post-traumatic stress disorder (PTSD).[98] Social anxiety disorder, for example, is often paired with abuse of alcohol and sedatives such as barbiturates.[99]

One study revealed that two-thirds of 102 alcoholic admissions to an alcohol treatment facility suffered from phobic symptoms, with one-third having agoraphobia or a social phobia. Other research demonstrated that in the majority of alcoholic phobics their phobias predated their alcohol dependence.[100]

Comorbidity compounds each problem. In addition to each exacerbating the other, the combination of substance abuse and an anxiety disorder or depression puts the person at greater risk of suicide.[101]

 For more about depression and anxiety, see my book *The Natural Medicine Guide to Depression* and *The Natural Medicine Guide to Anxiety* (both from Hampton Roads, 2003).

Creativity and Substance Abuse

The romanticization of the artist who abuses alcohol or drugs perpetuates the view that creativity and substance abuse are linked and traps many addicted artists into thinking that their talent will dry up when they dry out. The preponderance of substance abuse among creative people seems to lend credence to this view. The reality is that addiction has felled many brilliant writers, musicians, painters, and actors, either during their lives by interfering with their work or through bringing about their premature death. Either way, the world was deprived of their further contributions.

Jungian analyst and writer Linda Schierse Leonard, Ph.D., who battled with alcoholism herself, explores the issue in her book *Witness to the Fire: Creativity and the Veil of Addiction.* She concludes: "The relationship between addiction and creativity, as I see it, is not a causal one. Rather, there is a parallel process occurring in the psyche of the addict and the creative person. Both descend into chaos, into the unknown underworld of the unconscious. . . . But the addict is pulled down, often without choice, and is held hostage by addiction; the creative person *chooses* to go down into that unknown realm. . . ."[102]

19

It may be that the same forces that draw artists to the creative life draw them to substance abuse as well, or perhaps the emotional and psychological complexity of the creative process leads the artist to seek escape, relief, or transcendence through drugs or alcohol. Whatever the reason, romanticizing the contribution of addiction to creativity obscures the ugly reality of its physical, mental, spiritual, interpersonal, financial, and occupational toll.

The Medical History of Addiction

Humans have sought mind-altering substances throughout their history. In 4000 B.C., ancient Sumerians used opium. Chinese use of marijuana dates back to at least 2700 B.C. Peyote has been featured in religious ceremonies since the time of the Aztecs and likely longer. Throughout time, there have probably also been people who abused these drugs.

In more recent human history, society regarded excessive use of alcohol and drugs as a moral weakness or sin. Vestiges of this view persist today, despite the widely adopted model of addiction as a physiological disease. The disease model was actually proposed as early as 1804 when a Scottish physician wrote an essay propounding the concept of alcohol abuse as a physical disorder.[104] Both the church and the medical profession objected strenuously to this idea, and it wasn't until the mid 1800s that physicians began to treat inebriates in institutions devoted to the purpose.

It was another one hundred years, however, before the medical profession, as represented by the American Medical Association (AMA), officially declared in 1956 that alcoholism is a disease.[105] Despite the ruling, belief in the addict's weakness of character continued to pervade medical circles.

Famous Artists Who Had Substance Abuse Problems

Writers/Poets/Playwrights

Charles Baudelaire
William Burroughs
Truman Capote
Jean Cocteau
Samuel Taylor Coleridge
Thomas De Quincey
Feodor Dostoevsky
Dashiell Hammett
Jack Kerouac
Jack London
Eugene O'Neill
Edgar Allan Poe
Alexander Pushkin
Jean Rhys
Arthur Rimbaud
Dylan Thomas
Leo Tolstoy
Tennessee Williams

Painters

Toulouse Lautrec
Amadeo Modigliani
Edvard Munch
Jackson Pollock
Dante Gabriel Rossetti

Actors

John Barrymore
Richard Burton
John Cassavetes
Montgomery Clift
Troy Donahue
Judy Garland
John Gilbert
Veronica Lake
Bela Lugosi
Marilyn Monroe
Spencer Tracy
Robert Young

Comedians

John Belushi
Lenny Bruce
W. C. Fields

Singers/Musicians/Composers

Miles Davis
Jerry Garcia
Jimi Hendrix
Billie Holiday
Janis Joplin
Jim Morrison
Charlie Parker
Cole Porter
Elvis Presley

The Neurotransmitter Model

The advent of the pharmaceutical age brought research into brain activity, prompted by the effect of certain drugs on mental states and behavior. The psychiatric profession gradually turned from an emphasis on psychological causation to a focus on dysfunction in brain chemistry as the source of mental disorders, including addiction. Neurotransmitters, the brain's chemical messengers that enable communication between cells, became the subject of research and drug development aimed at manipulating brain chemistry.

The current conventional medical view is that addiction is a brain disorder caused by an imbalance or dysfunction in neurotransmitters. Research suggests that the problem may have its roots in genetics.[106]

All addictive substances and activities affect neurotransmitters, and these effects are the source of the associated "high." As noted previously, dopamine is thought to be the primary neurotransmitter involved in all addictions. Dopamine is the neurotransmitter that regulates pleasure. Its domain is satisfaction and euphoria. Anything that makes us feel good, including a compliment or a hug, elevates the dopamine in our brains. Scientists now regard dopamine as "the master molecule of addiction."[107] It is thought that addicts increase their usage or the amount they use in order to maintain the high levels of dopamine they have become habituated to through substance abuse.

Research on dopamine has nearly eliminated the formerly widely held view that some substances are addictive, while others are simply habit-forming, as in heroin versus cigarettes.[108] (As a side note, as recently as 1964, the Surgeon General of the United States held that cigarette smoking was not an addiction.[109]) According to the dopamine hypothesis, any substances that act on dopamine offer the potential for abuse.

Other neurotransmitters implicated in addiction vary according to substance type. For example, as discussed earlier in the section on alcohol, drinking acts on GABA (gamma-aminobutyric acid) and impedes the supply of tryptophan (the amino acid precursor to the neurotransmitter serotonin) to the brain, which interferes with serotonin production.

Serotonin is "the single largest brain system known."[110] Serotonin is another of the "feel good" neurotransmitters. In addition to influencing mood, it is involved in sensory perception and the regulation of sleep and pain, to name but a few of its numerous activities. Among the symptoms of serotonin deficiency are worry, anxiety, obsessions, compulsions, panic, phobias, insomnia, depression, and suicidal thoughts.[111]

GABA also has a large presence in the brain, being extant in 30 to 50 percent of brain synapses.[112] (A synapse is the gap between two nerve cells, or neurons, across which nerve impulses pass.) It operates to stop excess nerve stimulation, thereby exerting a calming effect on the brain. Symptoms of deficiency include a stressed and burned-out state, an inability to relax, and tense muscles.[113]

Alcohol and heroin and other opiates affect endorphins and enkephalins. Deficiencies in these natural painkilling neurotransmitters result in vulnerability to physical and emotional pain.

Conventional Medical Treatment Today

Current conventional medical treatment of addiction predominantly uses the Minnesota Model, developed by the Hazelden Foundation of Center City, Minnesota, in the 1940s and 1950s, which is based on Twelve-Step principles.

While Alcoholics Anonymous (AA) and other Twelve-Step programs espouse the view that alcoholism and other addictions are progressive diseases, most often likened to diabetes or cancer, they give little to no attention to the subject of physical treatment. "Working the steps" involves addressing the psychological, moral, and spiritual aspects of addiction. This seems an inherent contradiction. If you had diabetes or cancer, would you neglect to get medical treatment for the physical components of your illness?

If addiction is a physiological disease, why aren't Twelve-Step programs talking about imbalances in neurotransmitters and nutritional approaches to correcting those imbalances? (I focus here on biochemistry because it is conventional medicine's own explanation for addiction. As you will see in the next chapter, there are many other factors that can play a role in substance abuse.) Some might argue that Twelve-Step programs are support groups, not treatment providers. However, they disseminate a lot of information on addiction and lay out a model for recovery. So where is the physical aspect of the disease in this model and in the disseminated information?

The above observations are not to undercut the tremendous value of Twelve-Step programs in providing a support network for the recovering addict. But for them to promote the view that the disease of addiction cannot be cured is to ignore a whole area of treatment that is potentially of enormous benefit to the individual. And when at least 90 percent of those working in drug treatment have received training that positions the Twelve-Step programs as the best option available,[114] information to the contrary is not likely to reach those who need it.

Other approaches in the addiction field are Rational Recovery (a nonspiritual-based alternative to Twelve-Step programs), cognitive-behavioral therapy (which works to identify and change thought patterns and behaviors associated with substance abuse), and harm reduction (a method that does not demand abstinence but seeks to reduce the harm that results from drug use; needle exchange programs are one example of harm reduction). While each of these makes valuable contributions, they likewise fail to address the biochemistry of addiction.

The drug approach to treatment is problematic, given the established addictive patterns of the patients. Perhaps the most important argument against the use of antianxiety, antidepressant, and other pharmaceuticals as treatment for addiction, however, is that they are not a treatment. They do nothing to address the deeper causes.

The biochemical component of conventional medical treatment involves the use of drugs. Methadone is used by the majority of heroin addiction treatment programs, at a cost of about $500 million a year.[115] Valium has traditionally been used in alcohol detox, leaving many with another addiction to kick. Antidepressants and anxiolytics are prescribed for the depression and anxiety that often plague those in recovery. Antidepressants are also prescribed for sex addiction with the stated purpose that these drugs will treat mood symptoms and reduce sexual obsessions.[116] Addiction experts have a need for medications that can get addicts through the first few months of treatment when risk of relapse is highest, especially among cocaine users.

The drug approach to treatment is problematic, given the established addictive patterns of the patients. Perhaps the most important argument against the use of antianxiety, antidepressant, and other pharmaceuticals as treatment for addiction, however, is that they are *not* a treatment. They do nothing to address the deeper causes.

What factors are producing the depression and panic attacks in the recovering addict? If indeed a neurotransmitter imbalance is contributing both to the mood states and the addiction itself, what can be done to correct the imbalance, rather than attempt to mask it with drugs? What other factors might be operational in a particular individual's addiction? If no drug is inherently addictive, what within this person is contributing to the addiction?

Chapter 2 explores the many factors involved in addiction, which can serve as a starting point for answering these questions.

2 Causes, Contributors, and Influences

It is clear from the statistics on usage that the source of addiction does not lie in a particular substance but in the individual. Only ten to 20 percent of people who try cocaine, heroin, and alcohol, for example, end up fitting into the category of substance abusers, and even fewer meet the criteria for addiction.[117] Other sources place the percentage of drinkers who are alcoholic at ten percent.[118] That still leaves 90 percent of drinkers unplagued by alcoholism. As for addiction to nicotine, there are 40 million people in the United States who have been able to give up smoking, and 90 percent of those who quit manage to do so on their own.[119] The fact that people become addicted to activities such as gambling or pornography viewing is further evidence that the chemical composition of a substance is not the source of addiction.

So what is it in millions of people around the world that leads them to develop an addiction?

Though addiction is still classified as a mental disorder, the prevailing model holds that its origin is biological rather than psychological; that is, that a brain dysfunction of some kind is the cause. This may be the prevailing model, but conventional medicine has yet to come up with a treatment for this cause. This model of addiction is also problematic in that it fails to explore other factors that may be contributing to or exacerbating addiction. A holistic medical model does not look to a single cause of addiction but regards it as a combination of biological, energetic, and psychospiritual factors that must be addressed in treatment for recovery to be long lasting.

While successful treatment depends on addressing the underlying factors in each individual, the worldwide epidemic of addiction suggests that shared environmental factors are operational. Environmental in this usage simply means not genetic, so toxins, nutritional deficiencies from a poor diet, and psychological and social pressures, for example, all fall in the environmental category. Though genetics may leave an individual vulnerable to developing addictions, environmental stressors likely play a role in tipping the balance toward addiction.

There is no doubt that modern life exposes us to

14 Factors in Addiction

The following factors can contribute to addiction:

1. Genetic vulnerability
2. Neurotransmitter deficiencies or dysfunction
3. Nutritional deficiencies and imbalances
4. Hypoglycemia and carbohydrate/sugar dysmetabolism
5. Allergies
6. Intestinal dysbiosis
7. Hormonal imbalances
8. Chemical toxicity
9. Mercury toxicity
10. Medical conditions
11. Stress
12. Other lifestyle factors
13. Energy imbalances
14. Psychological, spiritual, and social issues

multiple stressors, from the toxins in our food, air, water, and soil to the hectic pace, isolation, and spiritual emptiness of the technological age. We obviously can't eliminate all of our environmental stressors, but we can take steps to reduce our load. While it may not be possible to determine a direct causal link between an individual's addiction and the environmental factors present in that person's life, when the condition is resolved by identifying and removing or ameliorating those factors, it is safe to say that one or more of them was implicated. It is important to know that the combination of factors differs and the specifics of each factor vary from person to person because no two people have the exact same constitution or emotional and psychological makeup.

This chapter looks at 14 factors that can contribute to or influence addiction in some way. While the individual factors may seem to be predominantly physical, psychological, or spiritual in nature, keep in mind that each has reverberating effects on the other levels because body, mind, and spirit are integrally linked.

The approach of identifying and addressing underlying imbalances has far-reaching benefits for your health in general. Many of the factors discussed in this chapter contribute to a range of disorders in addition to addiction. Reducing the total burden of stressors in your life is a wise strategy for preventing illness.

1. Genetic Vulnerability

Much of the genetic research on addiction has focused on alcoholism. Studies have shown that alcoholism runs in families. The risk of becoming an alcoholic is four times greater among sons of alcoholic fathers than among sons of nonalcoholic fathers (female offspring do not seem to be as affected).[120] At the same time, most of the children of alcoholics do not become alcoholics themselves,[121] more than half of alcoholics have no family history of alcoholism,[122] and identification of an "alcoholic gene" has so far eluded scientists.

The current genetic theory of addiction relates to neurotransmitters (the brain's chemical messengers), specifically the dopamine system in the brain. As noted in chapter 1, scientists view the neurotransmitter dopamine as "the master molecule of addiction." The dopamine theory holds that low levels in the brain, which may be the result of a genetic abnormality, predispose a person to seek substances that raise the levels.[123]

Kenneth Blum, Ph.D., a researcher, author, and international authority on psychopharmacology (the science of the effects of drugs on behavior and emotions) and substance abuse, states: "Forty years of research into the causes of alcoholism and other addictions have led to one conclusion: Irresistible craving is a malfunction of the reward centers of the brain. . . . Genetic research . . . indicates that the malfunction begins in the gene."[124]

More specifically, the malfunction occurs in what Dr. Blum terms the "Brain Reward Cascade." This is the harmonious functioning of the brain's neurotransmitters, which work together in complex ways, to ensure the proper levels and function of dopamine in the

> ## In Their Own Words
>
> *"'Percocet did nothing for me,' I've been amazed to hear people say. Percocet did everything for me; that's why I took more and more."*
>
> —Cindy R. Mogil, author of *Swallowing a Bitter Pill*[128]

brain's reward center. (If you recall from chapter 1, pleasurable activities or occurrences, even something as simple as receiving a compliment, result in the release of dopamine in the brain, the "reward" or feel-good neurotransmitter.) Dr. Blum's research indicates that an anomaly in a dopamine receptor gene causes what he terms "the addictive brain." Receptors are the components of the nerve cell that receive the neurotransmitter.

According to Dr. Blum's model, the genetic defect results in a breakdown in the Brain Reward Cascade, which results in turn in a state of uneasiness and anxiety. This uncomfortable state prompts the person to look for amelioration through substances or behavior. Dr. Blum uses the phrase "Reward Deficiency Syndrome (RDS)" to refer to this "common genetic predisposition to addiction."[125]

Other research suggests that, in the case of alcoholism, there may be a genetic abnormality in the way the liver processes alcohol that predisposes a person toward alcoholism.[126]

Even if genetic factors linked to addiction are conclusively identified, genetics are not destiny. As one biochemical researcher stated, "Genetics doesn't mean hopeless or incurable. What genetics means, to me, is chemistry. Chemistry can be adjusted and corrected."[127] Dr. Blum's research supports this assertion, as he has found that supplementing with amino acids, the building blocks of neurotransmitters, can alleviate the Reward Deficiency Syndrome (see the following section).

While you may not be able to change your genetic inheritance, you have control over the environmental factors that may be contributing to your addiction. The first step is to identify these factors. Then you can take the appropriate measures to reduce or eliminate their influence.

2. Neurotransmitter Deficiencies or Dysfunction

As noted, according to the current theory of addiction, neurotransmitter deficiencies or dysfunction are the root of the problem and are likely caused by genetic factors. However, there are numerous environmental factors that can disturb neurotransmitter supply and function, from poor diet to toxins to energy imbalances. Many of the factors covered in this chapter can throw off brain chemistry. Focusing on genetics to the exclusion of environmental influences omits factors over which substance abusers can exert some control and ignores what should be regarded as vital aspects of addiction treatment.

The neurotransmitters most implicated in addiction are dopamine, GABA (gamma-aminobutyric acid), serotonin, endorphin, and enkephalin (see chapter 1 for a detailed discussion). As the research of Dr. Blum and other scientists indicates, the level of dopamine in particular in the brains of those who become addicted may be lower than normal. Imbalances in other neurotransmitters are also implicated as part of the Brain Reward Cascade (see previous section). Even if genetic vulnerability was responsible for the initial imbalances that led the person to seek relief in drugs or alcohol, substance abuse exacerbates the problem, further skewing neurotransmitter activity in the brain. For example, alcohol initially stimulates neurotransmitter release and then, with chronic drinking, causes a deficiency in or reduces the action of dopamine, serotonin, GABA, endorphin, and enkephalin.[129]

Natural medicine uses amino acids (delivered orally or intravenously; see chapter 3) to correct neurotransmitter deficiencies and support their proper functioning. The fact that depression, anxiety, withdrawal symptoms, and addictive cravings are reduced or eliminated by this method indicates that skewed biochemistry is a factor in addiction. Perhaps the cause is as simple as a deficiency of amino acids (see the following section). If the mechanism that threw the neurotransmitters out of balance to begin with is not purely on the biochemical level, however, then correcting the biochemistry will likely produce only temporary results, unless the therapy is continued as a maintenance measure.

 For more on neurotransmitters, see chapters 1 and 3.

For example, if there is a genetic tendency toward low dopamine, this may explain why some individuals need to continue taking amino acids on a long-term basis to maintain the benefits. Or there may be an energy interference or a psychospiritual factor (see the sections to follow) that is throwing off the brain chemistry. Until that factor is addressed, the biochemical correction will not hold. Conversely, treating the root problem, whether physical, energetic, psychological, or spiritual, often results in the neurotransmitter deficiency or dysfunction self-correcting as the body's innate ability to heal is restored.

3. Nutritional Deficiencies and Imbalances

Most substance addicts suffer from malnourishment, both because their diet is generally poor and because drugs and alcohol deplete nutrients. Their nutritional problems may have begun before their addiction, as nutritional deficiencies, notably of amino acids, vitamin-B complex, and zinc, have been linked to addictive cravings.[130] As nutritional deficiencies and imbalances both contribute to and result from substance abuse, their relationship to addiction is a vicious circle.

Amazingly, most recovery programs and the psychiatric profession in general do not address nutritional factors in the treatment of addiction. Even with the view of addiction as a biological brain disorder, nothing is done to supply the brain with its most basic fuel. Even with the knowledge that drugs and alcohol deplete nutrients, nothing is done to restore these nutrients. This glaring omission continues despite evidence of the benefits of nutritional intervention in all aspects of substance recovery, from easing withdrawal to a greater likelihood of staying off the substance.

One study of inpatient alcoholism treatment compared the results of adding a nutritional component to a standard program with the standard program alone. The nutritional component consisted of large doses of vitamins and minerals along with a dietary protocol. The study found that 81 percent of those who received the nutritional component had maintained their sobriety six months later, while only 33 percent of those in the standard program alone had done so.[131]

The resistance of the conventional recovery field to nutritional treatment has a long history. Most people do not know that Bill W. (Bill Wilson; in keeping with the respect for anonymity that is basic to AA meetings, its founder is widely referred to as Bill W.) toward the end of his life tried without success to get Alcoholics Anonymous, the immensely influential organization he had cofounded, to disseminate vital information on the need for vitamin therapy, particularly niacin supplements, in alcohol recovery.[132]

He had discovered the work of Abram Hoffer, M.D., Ph.D., a pioneer in the use of vitamin therapy to treat alcoholism and schizophrenia, and been impressed by the results he was achieving. Bill W. began taking niacin himself and found that it relieved the depression that had been such a chronic problem for him.

Current Alcoholics Anonymous literature states: "We in AA believe there is no such thing as a cure for alcoholism. We can never return to normal drinking, and our ability to stay away from alcohol depends on maintaining our physical, mental, and spiritual health. This we can achieve by going to meetings regularly and putting into practice what we learn there."[133]

 For more about the work of Dr. Hoffer, see my book *The Natural Medicine Guide to Schizophrenia* (Hampton Roads, 2003).

Dr. Hoffer reports that Bill regarded niacin "as completing the third leg of the stool, the physical to complement the spiritual and emotional."[134]

While his focus on niacin may have been somewhat narrow, it was a start. Unfortunately, as noted in chapter 1, the physical component is still missing from AA and other Twelve-Step programs, an unfortunate omission given the huge benefits to be gained from simple supplements.

It is important to note that these supplements are natural nutrients required by the body for health, and taking them need not raise concerns about creating another substance addiction. As Julia Ross, M.A., states in chapter 3, when the body no longer needs amino acids, for example, the effects change and the person often doesn't feel good taking them.

The nutritional deficiencies often implicated in substance abuse are amino acids, vitamin-B complex, vitamin C, calcium, magnesium, zinc, and certain essential fatty acids. While many people who abuse substances suffer from the same deficiencies, no two people have exactly the same nutritional profile. Blood chemistry analysis can determine the precise status of your nutrient levels. With this information, therapeutic intervention can then be tailored to your specific needs. Random supplementation may not address those needs and may even contribute to further skewing of nutrient ratios.

Amino Acids: The production of neurotransmitters requires the presence of certain amino acids or precursors. For example, tryptophan is the amino acid precursor for serotonin; L-phenylalanine and L-tyrosine are the precursors for dopamine and norepinephrine; and D-phenylalanine and DL-phenylalanine are the precursors for endorphins and enkephalins. (GABA is an amino acid that also acts as a neurotransmitter.)

Amino acids are the basic building blocks of protein. The body does not manufacture most of the amino acids it requires, so they must be obtained through protein in the diet. With a deficient diet or a genetic defect, the body is not able to produce sufficient neurotransmitters. As noted previously, neurotransmitter problems are implicated in addiction. The fact that withdrawal symptoms, addictive cravings, depression, and anxiety are reduced or eliminated by amino acid supplementation supports this. The depression and anxiety that persist after a person gives up drugs or alcohol are often the impetus for relapse. As you will learn in chapter 3, by rebalancing brain chemistry, amino acids can resolve these mood disturbances and lower the relapse rate.

Although supplementation may not address the root cause of amino acid deficiency, such as a protein-poor diet or genetic defect, it can correct the problem, unlike drugs that attempt to manipulate brain chemistry. It also increases the supply of neurotransmitters naturally, by simply supplying the body with the building materials it needs, instead of forcing the brain and the neurotransmitters into unnatural function to keep the neurotransmitters available. Further, amino acid supplementation is safe and far less expensive than prescription drugs.

Research into the application of amino acids in the treatment of addiction shows promising results. In one double-blind placebo-controlled study of 62 people in an inpatient program, the group given amino acids did better during withdrawal, showed less stress according to a physiological measure, scored higher on the BESS (behavioral, emotional, social, spiritual) test, and had one-sixth as many absences against medical advice as the placebo group.[135] Chapter 3 is devoted to a full discussion of amino acids.

Vitamins and Minerals: While substance abuse can result in a deficiency in a range of vitamins and minerals, common depletions are of the vitamin B family, including folic acid; vitamin C; and the minerals zinc, calcium, and magnesium.[136]

The B vitamins are vital to neurotransmitter function. Vitamin B_1 (thiamine), for example, is known as the "morale vitamin" due to the effects it exerts on mental state and the nervous system.[137] Vitamin B_1 is also necessary for carbohydrate metabolism, impairment of which may be operational in addiction, as discussed in the following section. Among its other functions, vitamin B_3 (niacin and niacinamide) helps maintain blood sugar levels, a factor in the hypoglycemia associated with addiction, also covered in the next section. Vitamin B_5 (pantothenic acid) is called the "anti-stress" vitamin because of its essential role in adrenal gland function (see Hormonal Imbalances).

Like the other B vitamins, vitamin B_6 (pyridoxine) is vital for normal brain function and aids in more body functions than any other nutrient.[138] Folic acid, a member of the B-vitamin family, aids in the manufacture of brain neurotransmitters and can be useful in treating depression. As B vitamins work together and in ratio, it is important when supplementing to make sure that you get the full vitamin B complex.

Among its many activities, vitamin C is necessary for immune and adrenal gland function. It is also a potent detoxifier that has a long history of use in reversing drug highs quickly, easing withdrawal, and reducing cravings.[139] Janice Keller Phelps, M.D., a specialist in the nutritional approach to addiction treatment, cites vitamin C as "perhaps the best and safest detoxifier known" and an essential ingredient in addiction treatment.[140]

Among the other nutrients Dr. Phelps uses to ease the withdrawal process are niacinamide for its antidepressant effects, pantothenic acid (vitamin B_5) for adrenal support, and calcium for its calming effects.[141]

Sufficient levels of calcium and magnesium are necessary for proper nerve function. Deficiencies in these minerals have been linked to anxiety. The mental symptoms of calcium deficiency strongly resemble those of an anxiety attack.[142] Magnesium is important in itself for nervous system health, and also because it is necessary for calcium metabolism and enhances the activity of vitamin B_6. Research has demonstrated that supplementation with the B vitamins, calcium, and magnesium has antianxiety effects.[143] You will learn in part 2 that anxiety is more than simply paired with addiction; it may be the motivating force behind the development of addiction, as people attempt to tranquilize their anxiety with substances and activities.

Zinc deficiency interferes with neurotransmitter function. GABA is a zinc-dependent neurotransmitter, and zinc works with vitamin B_6, which is directly involved in the production of other neurotransmitters.[144] As copper and zinc exist in ratio to each other, low zinc results in a relative excess of copper, which has been clearly linked to psychological problems, including paranoia.[145]

Many Americans suffer from low-grade nutritional deficiencies. Poor diet (notably the standard American diet of processed food) and malabsorption due to gastrointestinal dysfunction are common causes. The depleted mineral content of the soil in which crops are grown, which translates into food with a lower mineral content than our forebears enjoyed, is a factor as well. Many lifestyle practices and attributes of modern life deplete us of vitamins and minerals, regardless of how well we eat. These include stress, caffeine intake, pollution, and heavy metals such as the mercury in our dental fillings.

People who chronically abuse alcohol or drugs add that nutritional drain to all of the others. While food alone is unlikely to reverse the severe deficiencies often associated with addiction, it is a good health practice to ensure that your diet includes the foods that contain these nutrients. The following are dietary sources of the key nutrients discussed:

Vitamin B_1: brewer's yeast, wheat germ, sunflower seeds, soybeans, peanuts, liver and other organ meats

Vitamin B_3: brewer's yeast, rice bran, peanuts, eggs, milk, fish, legumes, avocado, liver and other organ meats

Vitamin B_6: brewer's yeast, wheat germ, bananas, seeds, nuts, legumes, avocado, leafy green vegetables, potatoes, cauliflower, chicken, whole grains

Vitamin B_{12}: liver, kidneys, eggs, clams, oysters, fish, dairy

Folic acid: brewer's yeast, leafy green vegetables, wheat germ, soybeans, legumes, asparagus, broccoli, oranges, sunflower seeds

Vitamin C: green vegetables (particularly broccoli, Brussels sprouts, green peppers, kale, turnip greens, and collards), fruits (particularly guava, persimmons, black currants, strawberries, papaya, and citrus; citrus contains less vitamin C than the other fruits)

Calcium: kale, turnip greens, collards, mustard greens, parsley, tofu, kelp, brewer's yeast, blackstrap molasses, cheese, egg yolk, almonds, filberts, sesame seeds, sardines

Magnesium: parsnips, tofu, buckwheat, beans, leafy green vegetables, wheat germ, blackstrap molasses, kelp, brewer's yeast, nuts, seeds, bananas, avocado, dairy, seafood

Zinc: oysters, herring, sunflower seeds, pumpkin seeds, lima beans, legumes, soybeans, wheat germ, brewer's yeast, dairy

Essential Fatty Acids: Research has discovered a link between lipids and mental disorders. Lipids are fats or oils, which are comprised of fatty acids. Lipids are necessary for the health of the blood vessels that feed the brain and comprise 50 to 60 percent of the brain's solid matter.[146] More specifically, nerve cells in the brain contain high levels of omega-3 essential fatty acids.[147]

Essential fatty acids (EFAs) are unsaturated fats (the kinds of fats that remain liquid at room temperature) that are required for many metabolic actions in the body. There are two main types: omega 3 and omega 6. The primary omega-3 EFAs are ALA (alpha-linolenic acid), found in flaxseed, canola oil, soybeans, and walnuts, and DHA (docosahexaenoic acid) and EPA (eicosapentaenoic acid), found in the oils of cold-water fish, such as salmon, mackerel, herring, and sardines. The primary omega-6 EFAs are linoleic acid or cis-linoleic acid, found in many vegetables and safflower, sunflower, corn, peanut, and sesame oils, and GLA (gamma-linolenic acid), found in evening primrose, black currant, and borage oils.

Chronic alcohol abuse is known to deplete DHA,[148] while GLA has been successfully used to minimize alcohol withdrawal symptoms and lift depression,[149] indicating that a deficiency may be operational.

One Scottish study by a pioneer in essential fatty acid research, English physician David Horrobin, found that when alcoholics with EFA levels 50 percent below normal were given EFA replacement in treatment, their withdrawal symptoms were significantly reduced, and 83 percent were still sober and free of depression a year later. This was in sharp contrast to the placebo subjects (subjects receiving an inactive substance without their being aware that it is inactive) who were equally deficient in EFAs. In their case, they suffered the usual withdrawal symptoms, and only 28 percent had not returned to drinking within a year.[150]

Research suggests that certain alcoholics (notably those with a Scottish, Welsh, Irish, Scandinavian, or Native American heritage) may have a genetic defect in the conversion in the brain of essential fatty acids to prostaglandins (hormonelike substances) that help prevent depression and overexcitability, among other functions. Research also indicates that GLA supplementation can help correct this problem.[151]

While heritage may be a factor, the standard American diet contributes to EFA deficiencies. A high consumption of hydrogenated oils is part of the problem. Hydrogenated oils (which are oils processed to extend shelf life) take up the fatty acid receptor sites in the body and interfere with normal fatty acid metabolism. Hydrogenated oils, also known as trans-fatty acids, are found in margarine, commercial baked goods, crackers, cookies, and other products. It is a good health practice for everyone to avoid hydrogenated oils and is of particular importance for those who already have an EFA deficiency or perhaps a defect in their EFA processing mechanisms.

4. Hypoglycemia and Carbohydrate/Sugar Dysmetabolism

Hypoglycemia is a deficiency of sugar (glucose) in the blood. Glucose is a product of the breakdown of carbohydrates during digestion and is a fundamental source of fuel for the brain. Blood sugar is kept level by insulin, which is released by the pancreas and aids cells in absorbing glucose. When the pancreas overproduces insulin, as happens in hypoglycemia, blood sugar levels plummet, and the brain is deprived of fuel. The symptoms associated with hypoglycemia include fatigue, depression, anxiety, irritability, restlessness, insomnia, and mental disturbances.

In the 1960s, hypoglycemia was proposed as a cause of addiction. As with the role of nutritional deficiencies, resistance to this view continues today despite numerous studies demonstrating that problems in carbohydrate/sugar metabolism are at least present in addiction, if not a precipitating factor. The intense sugar cravings that substance abusers experience after quitting drugs or alcohol lend further support to the connection.

Clinical psychologist James R. Milam, Ph.D., whose work with addiction was instrumental in shifting the paradigm of alcoholism from the psychological to the physiological, states that 95 percent of early- and late-stage alcoholics have erratic blood sugar levels, as demonstrated by a glucose tolerance test, which measures a person's ability to metabolize glucose.[152] Erratic blood sugar levels indicate a problem in sugar metabolism. "[A]n unstable blood sugar level often leads to an impulse to drink if not an outright conscious craving for alcohol," Dr. Milam notes.

While running a chemical-dependency program in the late 1970s, Joan Mathews Larson, Ph.D., discovered through glucose tolerance testing that 75 percent of the clients were hypoglycemic. She went on to found the Health Recovery Center (HRC) in Minneapolis, a landmark alcoholism treatment facility where treatment is based on biochemical repair, the natural restoration of brain and body chemistry. Random testing of HRC clients revealed that 88 percent were hypoglycemic. In addition, 91 of the 100 clients had extremely low levels of chromium, a trace mineral (a mineral found in minute quantities in food and tissue) that is vital for proper sugar metabolism.[153]

Clinical psychologist James R. Milam, Ph.D., whose work with addiction was instrumental in shifting the paradigm of alcoholism from the psychological to the physiological, states that 95 percent of early- and late-stage alcoholics have erratic blood sugar levels, as demonstrated by a glucose tolerance test, which measures a person's ability to metabolize glucose.

The HRC program, which includes controlling hypoglycemia through diet and supplements, results in a more than 74-percent recovery rate, according to Dr. Larson.[154] This is far above the 15 to 30 percent rate of recovery from alcoholism claimed by conventional approaches.

Alcohol is a simple carbohydrate, meaning that it is broken down into glucose quickly, as opposed to complex carbohydrates such as whole grains, which are broken down more slowly. Refined sugar, as found in sweets such as candy, cake, and cookies, soft drinks, and other sugared beverages, is also a simple carbohydrate. Cravings for alcohol and sugar are the starving brain's way of getting a quick fix of the fuel it needs.

Dr. Janice Phelps's work in addiction treatment led her to the conclusion that sugar dysmetabolism (problems with the metabolism of sugar in the body), which causes sugar cravings and sugar addiction, is at the root of all addictions. Addiction to street drugs, prescription drugs, alcohol, and nicotine all come from the same basic physiological flaw, as these substances temporarily satisfy the sugar craving, she says. "Underlying this addictiveness, I am convinced, is a biochemical error of carbohydrate metabolism," states Dr. Phelps. "If you are an addictive person, your body simply doesn't handle sugars the way other people's bodies do. No one has yet discovered exactly where the basic error lies."[155]

As noted in chapter 1, research has found that high intake of fat and sugar can actually disturb brain chemistry and lead to addictive cravings for these substances. Refined sugar also depletes the body of chromium, which as noted above is needed for sugar metabolism. So perhaps poor diet is sufficient to set the stage for addiction. Or perhaps the dysmetabolism stems from other causes, such as allergies or a pancreatic problem. It may be genetic or environmental or a combination of both. Further research is needed to confirm the range of sources from which sugar/carbohydrate dysmetabolism stems.

It is not necessary to await research results before proceeding with treatment. Implementing a hypoglycemic diet and avoiding caffeine and refined sugars help stabilize blood sugar and control sugar and other addictive cravings. A hypoglycemic diet emphasizes foods that are low on the glycemic index, meaning that they help keep blood sugar stable. These foods include fresh vegetables, protein, and certain complex carbohydrates. Foods that are high on the glycemic index, such as refined sugar products, boost the blood sugar level. As difficult as it is for recovering addicts, avoiding caffeine and sugar foods is very important. The spikes and plummets in blood sugar levels that these substances produce increase alcohol and drug cravings.

Niacin, pantothenic acid, chromium, magnesium, vitamin C, and the amino acid glutamine are supplements that can also help reduce cravings.[156] As noted previously, random supplementation is not the optimum approach, however. Working with a qualified healthcare professional to design a supplement program that fits your individual needs is likely to produce the best results.

5. Allergies

Until recently, allergies were thought to affect only the mucous membranes, the respiratory tract, and the skin. A growing body of evidence indicates that an allergy can have profound effects on the brain and, as a result, behavior. An allergy or intolerance that affects the brain is known as a brain allergy or a cerebral allergy. Such allergies produce a wide range of symptoms and conditions, including anxiety, depression, and other mental disorders. The changes in mood and behavior indicate that brain chemistry is altered. Allergies, then, can be another source of neurotransmitter imbalance.

In Dr. Larson's study of 100 clients with alcoholism, testing revealed that 73 percent had food allergies, with the most common being to wheat and dairy.[157] Allergies are not limited to food, however, but can be to virtually anything. Many people are not aware that they are suffering from allergies, as the symptoms are often not clearly linked with ingestion of a food or exposure to a problem substance, as is the case when someone experiences a dangerous constriction of their air passages after eating shellfish or breaks out in a rash after using a certain kind of soap.

Addictive cravings can be a symptom of an allergy. There are two responses to an allergen (allergy-causing substance): you can seek to avoid the substance or you can crave the very substance to which you are allergic. An allergy to sugar, for example, can underlie the sugar cravings discussed in the previous section. As you will learn in chapter 4, an allergy to tobacco can be fueling a smoking addiction, and an allergy to cocaine can be behind the craving for that drug. When allergies are implicated, their elimination can result in a cessation of the cravings.

Some addiction specialists regard addiction as a problem of an intolerance or allergy to the drug, alcohol, or other substance involved, due to a metabolic difference in the way the body handles these substances. As one such physician states, "I have personally come to view alcoholism basically as an adverse drug reaction that occurs not to everyone, but to those with a genetic predisposition to it."[158] When an addiction is resolved with the clearing of allergies, as demonstrated in chapter 4, it is safe to assume that allergies played a part.

When it comes to food allergies, they may actually be intolerances or sensitivities resulting from compromised immune and digestive systems. Once these factors are eliminated or eased, the food intolerances may disappear.

Food intolerances occur when the body doesn't digest food

adequately, which results in large undigested protein molecules entering the intestines from the stomach. When poor digestion is chronic, these large molecules push through the lining of the intestines, creating the condition known as leaky gut, and enter the bloodstream. There, these substances are out of context, not recognized as food molecules, and so are regarded as foreign invaders.

The immune system sends an antibody (also called an immunoglobulin) to bind with the foreign protein (antigen), a process which produces the chemicals of allergic response. The antigen-antibody combination is known as a circulating immune complex, or CIC. Normally, a CIC is destroyed or removed from the body, but under conditions of weakened immunity, CICs tend to accumulate in the blood, putting the body on allergic alert, if you will. Thereafter, whenever the person eats the food in question, an allergic reaction follows. The digestive dysfunction inherent in food allergies can affect the brain, as discussed in the next section.

The subject of allergies and addiction is explored thoroughly in chapter 4.

6. Intestinal Dysbiosis

In addition to food allergies and the problems in the metabolism or digestive breakdown of carbohydrates discussed previously, other factors can affect digestive function, which in turn can disturb brain biochemistry.

One such factor is intestinal dysbiosis, which means an imbalance of the flora that normally inhabit the intestines. Among these flora are the beneficial bacteria (known as probiotics) *Lactobacillus acidophilus* and *Bifidobacterium bifidum,* potentially harmful bacteria such as *E. coli* and *Clostridium,* and the yeastlike fungus *Candida albicans.* Habitual drinking, anti-inflammatory drugs, antibiotics, food allergies, and a poor diet can all contribute to disturbing the balance among these flora.

When the balance is disturbed, the microorganisms held in check by the beneficial bacteria proliferate and release toxins that compromise intestinal function. This has far-reaching effects in the body and on the mind. Research has revealed that what passes through the lining of the intestines (see Allergies) can make its way through the bloodstream to the brain.[159]

Anxiety, depression, and fatigue are three of the most common effects of an intestinal overgrowth of *Candida*.[160] The fungus, through its normal metabolic processes, releases substances that are toxic to the brain and interfere with neurotransmitter activity.[161] In addition, with an overgrowth, the intestinal lining becomes inflamed, which interferes with the absorption of nutrients.[162] As discussed earlier, nutritional deficiencies contribute to neurotransmitter imbalance and can play a role in addiction.

With the particularly close link between addiction and anxiety in particular, it is important to consider the contribution of intestinal dysbiosis to anxiety. Gastrointestinal complaints such as diarrhea, constipation, gas, and stomach pains are common in anxiety disorders. A survey of over 13,000 people with panic disorder, for example, revealed that the rate of gastrointestinal symptoms was significantly higher among them than in the general population.[163] While it may be difficult to determine whether these symptoms are a cause or a consequence of anxiety, the relationship between anxiety and intestinal dysbiosis is clearly another vicious circle situation, with each condition worsening the other.

There is also a direct link between intestinal dysbiosis and alcoholism. Among the factors that contribute to *Candida* overgrowth are excessive intake of sugar, carbohydrates, and alcohol, as the fungus feeds on sugar. Dr. Larson found that 25 percent of her sample of 100 Health Recovery Center clients had *Candida* overgrowth. Another study of 213 HRC clients revealed that this condition was present in 55 percent of the women and 35 percent of the men.[164]

Candida overgrowth occurs when something intervenes to disturb the normal balance of flora in the intestinal environment. In addition to excess intake of sugar, carbohydrates, and alcohol, other factors that can contribute to *Candida* overgrowth are excessive use of antibiotics; a chlorinated drinking water supply; exposure to heavy metals such as mercury, pesticides, and other chemicals; a nutrient-poor diet; and hormonal treatment (hormone replacement, birth control pills, cortisone).[165]

Eliminating foods that "feed" *Candida* is a common treatment approach to restoring intestinal balance. The so-called Candida diet emphasizes avoiding all forms and sources of sugar, including fruit and fruit juice, carbohydrates, and fermented yeast products—and naturally, alcohol. Taking a probiotic supplement (acidophilus and other "friendly" bacteria) can also help restore the balance of intestinal flora.

A number of natural medicine practitioners, notably Thomas M. Rau, M.D., director of the Paracelsus Klinik in Lustmühle, Switzerland, have discovered the connection between *Candida* and mercury, postulating that one of the functions of the fungus in the body is to deal with heavy metals such as mercury, for which it has a particular affinity. If there is a high level of mercury in the body, *Candida* multiplies. Until you detoxify the body of the mercury, says Dr. Rau, you won't be able to get rid of the *Candida* overgrowth on any lasting basis, no matter how perfect your diet or what antifungal drug or natural substance you take. The fungus will just keep coming back.[166]

The number of factors that enter a discussion of intestinal dysbiosis highlights the complex interrelationship between the conditions that can cause or contribute to addiction. Sugar metabolism problems, allergies, intestinal dysbiosis, nutritional deficiencies, and mercury toxicity can each impact on the other, and it's impossible to separate the causes from the consequences. This reality supports the logic of a multimodal approach to the treatment of addiction.

7. Hormonal Imbalances

Hormones are "probably second only to the chemicals of the brain in shaping how we feel and behave."[167] Hormonal imbalances influence brain chemistry and the nervous system. Organic dysfunction, hormonal treatment, toxic exposure, stress, diet, and exercise can all affect hormonal levels and balance. Chronic alcohol abuse can also disrupt hormonal balance.[168] Adrenal gland, thyroid gland, and reproductive hormones can play a role in addiction.

Research indicates that people with addiction problems may have a malfunction in what is known as the hypothalamic-pituitary-adrenal axis.[169] This is a system of hormones that regulate carbohydrate metabolism, blood sugar level, appetite, emotions, desires, urges, and a sense of well-being, among other functions.

Dopamine is among the hormones released by the hypothalamus, a supervisory center in the brain. The pituitary gland, located at the base of the brain, releases the hormones vasopressin and ACTH (adrenocorticotrophic hormone), which are involved in stress response. Vasopressin constricts blood vessels, causing blood pressure to rise, and ACTH stimulates the adrenal glands to release the stress hormone cortisol, which is also involved in carbohydrate metabolism.

In addition to secreting cortisol, the two adrenal glands, which are situated one atop each kidney, synthesize and store dopamine and the stress hormones epinephrine (adrenaline) and norepinephrine (noradrenaline). Norepinephrine is similar to epinephrine and is the form of adrenaline found in the brain, where it functions as a neurotransmitter.[170] In addition to their involvement in the stress response, adrenaline and noradrenaline play a part in the physiology of fear and anxiety.

Research indicates that people with addiction problems may have a malfunction in what is known as the hypothalamic-pituitary-adrenal axis. This is a system of hormones that regulate carbohydrate metabolism, blood sugar level, appetite, emotions, desires, urges, and a sense of well-being, among other functions.

The adrenaline rush produced by stress, amphetamines, caffeine, and other stimulants contributes to the destabilization of blood sugar, as adrenaline prompts the liver to release glycogen (stored sugar), which in turn prompts the release of insulin to try to balance the increased blood sugar (see Hypoglycemia). With chronically low blood sugar, adrenaline must continue to be pumped into the bloodstream. Thus substance abuse, prolonged stress, and low blood sugar (hypoglycemia) exhaust the adrenal glands and disturb adrenal hormone balance. Habitual drinking depletes pantothenic acid (vitamin B_5), which is required in adrenal hormone production.[171]

The thyroid, a bow-shaped gland located in the throat region, regulates body temperature and energy use, among other functions. Thyroid hormone operates both as a hormone and as a neurotransmitter.

Substance abuse, of both stimulants and depressants, can affect the production of thyroid hormone. Hypothyroidism (an underactive thyroid gland) is common in nicotine addiction and alcoholism.[172] It is often overlooked, however, because it can be at a subclinical level, meaning standard tests fail to detect it. Over 50 percent of the estimated 13 million Americans who have thyroid disease are not aware of it.[173] Among the symptoms of hypothyroidism are fatigue, depression, and anxiety. More research is needed into the relationship between thyroid hormone and addiction, as the results could influence treatment approaches.

Reproductive hormones, particularly the "female" hormones estrogen and progesterone, may also be a factor in addiction. A condition called estrogen dominance, which is having too much estrogen in relation to progesterone, is often associated with addiction.[174] Interestingly, estrogen dominance also tends to manifest in anxiety.[175] Estrogen dominance has become more common as a result of what are known as environmental estrogens (xenoestrogens), ubiquitous chemical toxins that, once in the body, mimic the effects of estrogen. A deficiency of omega-3 essential fatty acids with a relative excess of omega-6 essential fatty acids is another factor that can cause estrogen dominance.[176] Natural progesterone, in an oral or cream form, can help restore a healthy ratio of progesterone to estrogen.

8. Chemical Toxicity

Humans today are exposed to an unprecedented number of chemicals. Testing of anyone on Earth, no matter how remote the area in which they live, will reveal that they are carrying at least 250 chemical contaminants in their body fat.[177] The effects of this toxic overload on the human body are only beginning to be investigated.

The Greater Boston Physicians for Social Responsibility released a report summarizing research on lead, mercury, cadmium, manganese, nicotine, pesticides (many of which are commonly used in homes and schools), dioxin and PCBs (polychlorinated biphenyls; both PCBs and dioxin stay in the food chain once they enter it, as they pervasively have), and solvents used in paint, glue, and cleaning products.

The report notes that in one year alone (1997), industrial plants released over a billion pounds of these chemicals directly into the environment (air, water, and land). Further, almost 75 percent of the top 20 chemicals (those released in the largest quantities) are known or suspected to be neurotoxicants.[178] (Neurotoxicants or neurotoxins are substances that are toxic to the brain and the nervous system in general.) Other sources report that of 70,000 different chemicals being used commercially only 10 percent have been tested for their effect on the nervous system.[179] In addition to the pesticides used directly on crops, the chemicals in the air, water, and soil are fully integrated into our food supply.

Chemicals to which we are regularly exposed can disturb the production and function of neurotransmitters, block their receptor sites (preventing the uptake of neurotransmitters and thus their vital function as the chemical messengers of the brain), and prevent enzymes (the specialized proteins required in every chemical reaction in the body) from working.[180] So, chemical toxicity must be added to the list of factors that can lead to neurotransmitter deficiencies or dysfunction, which is the underlying cause of addiction, according to the conventional medical model. Chemical exposure has been linked to alcoholic cravings and a higher risk of relapse.[181] Generally, the phrase "chemical toxicity," as it is used in natural medicine, does not signify acute poisoning by toxic chemicals, but to the toxic load the body carries as a result of chronic exposure to a range of chemicals over time.

As just one chemical, consider the hydrazines, a family of widely used chemicals, notably in pesticides, jet fuels, and growth retardants. Hydrazine is sprayed on potatoes to prolong their shelf life. In the body, this chemical blocks serotonin production by blocking the action of vitamin B_6, which is needed at every step in the series of enzyme actions required in the manufacture of serotonin. In just one bag of potato chips or one serving of fast-food French fries, there is sufficient hydrazine to knock out all the B_6 in your body.[182]

9. Mercury Toxicity

Heavy metal toxicity may also be a factor in addiction. As with chemical toxicity, research is needed to explore this link. The neurotoxicity of the heavy metal mercury, however, has been recognized for centuries. Early hatmakers contracted what was known as "mad hatter's disease," the result of poisoning from the mercury used in hatmaking, hence the saying "mad as a hatter."

Physiologically, mercury's effects on the brain arise from its ability to bond firmly with structures in the nervous system, explains Dietrich Klinghardt, M.D., Ph.D., whose work is featured in chapter 7. Research shows that mercury is taken up in the peripheral nervous system by all nerve endings (in the tongue, lungs, intestines, and connective tissue, for example) and then transported quickly via nerves to the spinal cord and brainstem.

"Once mercury has traveled up the axon, the nerve cell is impaired in its ability to detoxify itself and in its ability to nurture itself," says Dr. Klinghardt. "The cell becomes toxic and dies—or lives in a state of chronic malnutrition. . . . A multitude of illnesses, usually associated with neurological symptoms, result."[183]

Mercury is bioaccumulative, which means that it doesn't break down in the environment or in the body. The result is that it is everywhere in our environment, in our food, air, and water, and each exposure adds to our internal accumulation. Many of us also carry a source of mercury in our mouths in the form of dental fillings; so-called silver fillings are actually comprised of over 50 percent mercury. Scientific studies have shown that these fillings leach mercury, predominantly in the form of vapor, 80 percent of which is absorbed through the lungs into the bloodstream. Chewing raises the level of vapor emission and it remains elevated for at least 90 minutes afterward.[184]

Among the symptoms that improve after having mercury amalgam fillings replaced with nontoxic composite fillings are anxiety, nervousness, irritability, insomnia, depression, fatigue, lack of energy, headaches, memory loss, lack of concentration, allergies, gastrointestinal disturbance, and thyroid problems. The presence of mental, mood, and behavioral conditions lends further support to mercury's influence on the brain.

It is also interesting to note the overlap with the other factors implicated in addiction, notably allergies, gastrointestinal disturbance, and thyroid problems. As discussed previously, mercury toxicity can also contribute to nutritional deficiencies and *Candida* overgrowth (intestinal dysbiosis).

 For more about mercury, see chapter 7.

Hair analysis is one laboratory test used to determine mercury and other heavy metal levels in the body. It can be used to measure the level of both minerals and heavy metals, as these levels in the hair are an indicator of the overall levels in the body. For a more precise analysis of the body's level of mercury, a DMPS challenge test can be used. For this, the person is injected with the chelating agent DMPS (2,3-dimercaptopropane-1-sulfonate). Chelating means that the substance binds with heavy metals such as mercury and carries them out of the body via the urine. A urinalysis run after the chelating agent has had time to work then reveals what heavy metals are present in higher than normal levels in the body.

10. Medical Conditions

As discussed in this chapter and chapter 1, medical conditions frequently present in addiction include hypoglycemia (low blood sugar), allergies, *Candida* overgrowth, hypothyroidism (underactive thyroid gland), ADD (attention deficit disorder), clinical depression, and anxiety disorders such as obsessive-compulsive disorder, panic disorder, social anxiety disorder (social phobia), specific (simple) phobia, generalized anxiety disorder (GAD), and posttraumatic stress disorder (PTSD).

The conditions can both precede and exacerbate the addiction problem. Regarding the preponderance of anxiety disorders in addiction, clinical psychologist Roger J. Callahan, Ph.D., the founder of Thought Field Therapy and the author of *The Anxiety-Addiction Connection,* maintains that all addiction problems stem from an attempt to tranquilize anxiety (see chapter 8).

Psychopharmacology expert Kenneth Blum, Ph.D., and other proponents of amino acid therapy (see chapter 3) cite neurotransmitter problems as the source of both addiction and the mental conditions that accompany it, such as depression, anxiety, and ADD.

11. Stress

Stress is involved in addiction in a number of ways. Perhaps the most obvious connection is that people turn to substances or addictive activities for relief from stress. Cigarette smoking is a pervasive example. It is used by many smokers as a calming agent throughout the day and particularly during moments of upset or when they are in a stressful situation. Stress is also implicated in relapses that occur after quitting a substance. More than one-third of relapses arise from stress and the negative emotions associated with it.[185]

One illustration of the role of stress as an impetus for substance abuse is the widespread use of heroin among soldiers during the Vietnam War and the fact that once returned home and removed from that tremendously stressful situation, few continued using.[186]

Chronic stress also exhausts the adrenal glands (see Hormonal Imbalances), as do substance abuse and hypoglycemia. This further impairs the ability to cope with stress and sets up yet another vicious circle. Like substance abuse, chronic stress depletes the body of nutrients, which compromises the brain's neurochemistry and other body systems. Chronic stress can also throw off the balance of the energy system of the body (see Energy Imbalances), which can contribute to and exacerbate addiction. In fact, chronic stress exerts a tremendous strain on the body, mind, and spirit, creating a complex web of interacting factors that all support addiction.

The fact that stress is so interwoven with addiction is a strong argument for reducing the amount of stress in your life wherever possible, whether through avoidance of known stressful situations, making changes in your circumstances or lifestyle, and/or practicing meditation and relaxation techniques. In addition, attending to the other factors in this chapter can significantly reduce your stress load.

12. Other Lifestyle Factors

Twelve-Step programs offer a handy acronym as a reminder of some factors that can contribute to relapse: HALT! Don't get too **h**ungry, **a**ngry, **l**onely, or **t**ired. Added to that could be: avoid or reduce your intake of caffeine and get regular exercise.

Caffeine produces abrupt changes in blood sugar and exacerbates hypoglycemia, both of which contribute to addictive cravings.[187] As it sends adrenaline flowing through the body, excessive use can also contribute to adrenal depletion, which has a number of implications for addiction (see Hormonal Imbalances and Stress).

Caffeine does a lot more than give you a jittery edge. It actually affects your neurotransmitters, stimulating the release of norepinephrine and others. As with alcohol, habitual excess intake can leave you with a neurotransmitter deficit, along with hypoglycemia, and nutritional deficiencies, as caffeine interferes with the absorption of important nutrients such as B vitamins, magnesium, calcium, potassium, and zinc.[188] Note the overlap with deficiencies implicated in addiction (see Nutritional Deficiencies and Imbalances). In the general population, people who drink a lot of coffee test higher for anxiety and depression.[189]

Avoiding caffeine or at least limiting intake is thus advisable. Be sure to consider all caffeine sources. Some people give up or cut down on coffee and black tea but overlook the high caffeine content in colas.

Exercise stimulates the release of mood-regulating neurotransmitters, along with endorphins, which lift mood and reduce stress level. It increases oxygen, glucose, and nutrient supply to the brain, which improves cerebral function and the ability to cope with stress.[190] Exercise also helps flush toxins out of the body, the benefits of which have been discussed previously.

Exercise can alleviate anxiety, irritability, hyperactivity, insomnia, and depression,[191] all of which are associated with addiction. Along with proper nutrition and sleep, it is a basic need of the body. Lack of exercise is an environmental stressor that is relatively easy to remedy.

13. Energy Imbalances

As discussed in the section on neurotransmitters, an energy interference can throw off brain chemistry. There are a number of different ways to discuss the flow of energy in the human body from a natural medicine perspective. You could speak of the body's electromagnetic or energy field and the far-reaching effects on physical and mental health caused by disturbances in that field (see chapters 4 and 7). If you regard energy from the perspective of traditional Chinese medicine, which is an energy-based medicine, illness is regarded as a disturbance in the individual's *qi*, or vital energy (see chapters 4 and 5). If you consider energy from a psychic viewpoint, you might explore the presence of "foreign energy" (as it were, belonging to somebody or something else) in an individual's energy field (see chapter 9).

Developmental Stages and Addiction

Is there a relationship between the substance that a person abuses in later life and interference or blockage that occurred at a certain stage in that person's childhood development? Yes, according to Johannes Beckmann, M.D., a general practitioner who specializes in psychosomatic medicine and runs a private practice in Palma de Mallorca, Spain. Psychosomatic medicine is a European medical discipline that recognizes the role and interrelationship of body and mind in mental and physical health.

Blockage or interference prevents the child from progressing to the next stage of development. The blockage can be a deficit or excess of what the child needs at a certain stage. An example is too much or too little control at the movement stage (stage 3), which may prevent the child from moving on to the social-sexual stage (stage 4). Or the source of the interference can be a trauma of some kind at that stage, which prevents normal development, Dr. Beckmann explains. Finally, a person can be stuck at a certain stage by blockage at the next stage, which effectively keeps the child from moving on.

The impulses and needs of each childhood stage as defined in this model are experienced in later life through different addictions, says Dr. Beckmann. The following are the childhood development stages and the subsequent preferred substances or activities that are associated with interferences (blockages) at each stage.

1. **Blockage at the umbilical stage (intrauterine life):** interference from trauma in the later stages of intrauterine life (the longing to return to this stage necessitates an intrauterine experience that is largely one of security and well-being), birth trauma, or blockage of the oral stage (stage 2)
   Preferred substances: heroin, morphine, opium, hallucinogens

2. **Blockage at the oral stage (from birth through first year):** interference from deficit of or excessive breast-feeding, or blockage of the motoric stage (stage 3)

Preferred substances/activities: cigarettes, alcohol, chewing gum, food addiction, bulimia

3. **Blockage at the motoric or movement stage (from beginning to walk to two and a half years old):** what Freud terms the anal stage; interference from external influences that exert no control or too much control on the child's impulsivity, or blockage of the social-sexual stage (stage 4)
Preferred substances/activities: ecstasy, amphetamines, cocaine, steroids, body-building or sports addiction

4. **Blockage at the social-sexual stage (two and a half to four years old):** stage of taking one's position in the family, taking responsibility for one's actions; interference from lack of definition or confusion over role, being given too much or too little responsibility, or blockage of the sexual stage (stage 5)
Preferred activities: workaholism, addiction to psychological behavior patterns such as being a victim or an intimidator, pornography addiction

5. **Blockage at the sexual stage (four to seven years old):** what Freud terms the Oedipal stage
Preferred substances/activities: chocolate, sex and relationship addictions, repetitive patterns in relationships

Whatever language you choose to employ to describe the phenomenon, a disturbance in an individual's energy field can contribute to addiction. The relationship of energy to other factors can be cyclical, with physical factors (such as neurotransmitter dysfunction or nutritional deficiencies) or psychological or spiritual issues causing or being caused by a disturbance in energy flow. Most of the chapters in part 2 explain and explore in depth energy imbalances as a factor in addiction.

14. Psychological, Spiritual, and Social Issues

To ignore the psychological and spiritual factors in any illness is to treat only part of a person. As noted in the section on Energy Imbalances, psychological and spiritual issues have the capacity to throw the energy system out of balance, which can have repercussions on all levels, including neurotransmitter function. Thus, treatment that does not address all areas will not produce lasting health.

Exploring the psychological and spiritual dimensions of addiction does not mean a return to blaming addiction on a character flaw. It could be considered psychological and spiritual housecleaning or the maintenance work that taking good care of something requires. Taking good care of yourself means attending to the needs of your body, mind, and spirit. Chapters 6 to 9 offer different ways of exploring the psychological and spiritual components of addiction.

With addiction, social factors also play a significant role. With whom and how we choose to spend our time can perpetuate addiction or promote recovery. In addition, a social support system or the lack thereof has a profound effect. One study of 1,000 patients who had undergone conventional alcoholism treatment revealed that of the 28 percent who were still sober eight years later (though many relapsed at least once during that time), nearly all had a strong support system.[192]

Psychologist Stanton Peele, Ph.D., a specialist in the field of addiction, states, "[T]he crux of the struggle against addiction lies in the social and cultural environments we create."[193]

As a number of the physicians and other practitioners whose work is covered in part 2 state, the social component must be an adjunct to treatment that restores the balance of the body. This means establishing some kind of support network, whether through friends, family, a Twelve-Step program, or other addiction recovery support group, and avoiding a return after treatment to the social crowd and activities connected to one's substance abuse.

The social aspect of addiction extends far beyond the individual, however. Why is it that so many people in the world need to self-medicate? The toxicity of our world and the stress of modern living may be factors, but how else are our familial, community, political, and religious structures failing us? With addiction a worldwide epidemic, it cannot be viewed as a problem for individuals to solve for themselves. Yes, it is up to you to attend to the factors discussed in this chapter and work to reverse your own addiction, but the global epidemic is everyone's responsibility.

Action Plan

Based on the recommendations of the practitioners in this book and the scientific literature of addiction, the following are steps you can take to eliminate the causes, triggers, and contributors to your addiction.

- Eat a healthful, balanced diet; avoid caffeine and sugar.

- Consult with a qualified practitioner of natural medicine to identify any amino acid deficiencies and decide on oral supplements or intravenous treatment to correct them (see chapter 3). (A qualified practitioner is someone who has had advanced training in natural medicine and is well versed in the area of practice in which you require expertise, such as the use of amino acid supplements.)

- Have your biochemical status checked to identify any nutritional deficiencies or imbalances, and take the appropriate supplements to correct them (see chapters 3 and 7).

- Avoid foods and other substances to which you are allergic, or get allergy treatment such as NAET to eliminate the problem (see chapter 4). If you suspect you have allergies, but don't know to what, NAET can help you identify the allergens.

- Consult with a qualifed practitioner of natural medicine to determine if you have an overgrowth of *Candida*. Implement dietary measures and take probiotics to restore intestinal health.

- Have a qualified practitioner check you for hormonal imbalances.

- Reduce your toxic exposure wherever possible. Avoid using toxic house and garden products; eat organically grown food; and drink pure water instead of tap water.

- Reduce your mercury exposure wherever possible. You may want to investigate having your mercury dental fillings replaced with non-mercury amalgams; hair analysis and other tests can determine if the level of mercury in your body is high (see chapter 7).

- Work with your doctor to determine if you have any medical conditions implicated in addiction, such as hypothyroidism or hypoglycemia.

- Find ways to reduce or manage the stress in your life. Meditation and relaxation techniques can be beneficial.

- Get regular exercise.

- Address energy imbalances through acupuncture, flower essence therapy, or other forms of energy-based medicine (see chapters 5 and 6).

- Explore psychospiritual issues through psychotherapy or other modalities (see chapters 6–9).

PART II

Natural Medicine Treatments for Addiction

3 The Biochemistry of Addiction: Amino Acids and Neurotransmitter Restoration

Julia Ross, M.A., who holds a master's degree in clinical psychology, is a pioneer in the field of nutritional psychology and has 25 years of experience directing counseling programs that address addiction, mood problems, and eating disorders. Nutritional psychology recognizes the central role that biochemistry plays in mental health and regards nutritional intervention in the form of dietary changes and supplements as an essential treatment for restoring that health. The use of amino acids (the building blocks of proteins necessary in neurotransmitter production) is the centerpiece of her therapeutic approach to addiction recovery.

Ross developed this approach "out of desperation when we found that the conventional approach was just not working." Prior to that, however, she'd had great hopes for the standard psychological/spiritual approach. In the 1970s and 1980s, she was working in a large residential treatment program, conducting individual, family, and group therapy. Until the mid-eighties, most of the residents were alcoholics. The residents responded enthusiastically to the psychotherapy programs she and her colleagues had developed, which they used in combination with the Twelve-Step program.

"We wouldn't hear from these people after they graduated, but we assumed that everything was fine. How could it not be? They'd done so well, they'd loved it. Their families were so grateful, everybody was happy," recalls Ross.

In those days, addiction treatment had begun to attract a lot of attention, and researchers began to conduct follow-up studies on recidivism (relapse) rates. In 1986, Ross and her treatment colleagues all over the country got the results of the first studies. They were shocked to learn what was actually happening to the people they had thought had overcome their alcohol problems. Only 50 percent of them were still not drinking.

The missing piece in the treatment model was that it had failed to address addictive cravings and "inner mood states," Ross recalls. Despite the fact that the life circumstances of the people who had gone through the programs had dramatically improved, quitting alcohol had left them with depression and anxiety. "With this persistent, negative mood state, some of them actually felt worse in recovery than they had felt while they were drinking," she observes.

Understandably, Ross and her colleagues were disturbed by these results. They cast around for an explanation for the mood state. An obvious conclusion was that substance abuse masks emotional pain, but as residents of her program received extensive therapy to explore underlying psychological issues during a stay that lasted six months to two years, this was not a plausible reason.

At the same time that the research results revealed to Ross and her fellow counselors that they were failing to meet some of the needs of their alcoholic clients, they were facing a whole new population of substance abusers for whom their program was clearly not working. The mid-eighties had brought the crack cocaine epidemic, along with a sharp rise in the use of other kinds of cocaine. Among crack cocaine users, the relapse rate approached 100 percent, which was obvious by the nearly universal exodus mid-treatment with the same users returning a few months later to try again.

Ross realized that there was one area that treatment had been neglecting. While she and her colleagues covered the emotional, psychological, behavioral, and spiritual aspects of addiction thoroughly, they did very little to address the physical, as was true of conventional recovery in general. While Ross's and other residential programs provided three square meals a day, which was in most cases a vast dietary improvement for substance abusers, that was the extent of the physical component of treatment.

 For more about sugar cravings and addiction, see chapter 2.

As Ross began to research the physical component of addiction, information was just emerging in the scientific literature about the connection between relapse and physiological imbalances that affected mood, energy, and sleep. This confirmed what Ross had witnessed with cocaine and crack addicts in particular. At a certain point in treatment, they would hit what is known in cocaine recovery circles as "the wall." They would suddenly become so exhausted and depressed that it was untenable for them to continue with treatment. Having signed on for a 30-day program, they would disappear after ten or 15 days. This high rate of absences against medical advice was duplicated in cocaine addiction programs all over the country.

Ross had already instituted nutritional counseling as part of the treatment program, with the main recommendations being to avoid sugar and white flour, emphasize protein, and eat lots of vegetables, but had found that not many people could follow this regimen. Intense sugar cravings led to a high consumption of candy bars, desserts, and heavily sugared coffee, even when residents were aware that sugar and caffeine destabilized their moods and increased the likelihood of cravings for their former substance of choice, whether drugs or alcohol.

Fortunately, Ross came across the work of Kenneth Blum, Ph.D., a scientist specializing in the area of brain chemistry and addiction (see chapter 2). His explanation for addictive cravings as a largely genetic problem in the programming of the brain's mood chemistry via the neurotransmitters rang true for Ross. But more significantly, his research identified the missing piece in addiction recovery programs—amino acids.

"He paid attention to something that other scientists have wanted to ignore in the service of making money by developing drugs that manipulate brain chemistry," states Ross. "He paid attention to what all neuroscientists know, and that is that these unbelievably powerful natural mood-enhancing neurotransmitters are made out of amino acids, the building blocks of protein. Blum pointed out that if you identified which neurotransmitter was deficient in someone who was addicted and gave that person the amino acid that feeds that particular neurotransmitter production system, you could increase the level of that neurotransmitter within days."

The amino acid precursors of the primary neurotransmitters implicated in addiction are as follows:

Neurotransmitter	Amino Acid Precursor
Serotonin	tryptophan; 5-HTP
Norepinephrine/dopamine	L-tyrosine; L-phenylalanine
Endorphins, enkephalins	D-phenylalanine; DL-phenylalanine
GABA	GABA

Within a month of reading about Dr. Blum's findings, Ross introduced amino acid therapy at the treatment center. The results were startlingly immediate. The most significant changes were dramatic reductions in anxiety and depression and, amazingly, the complete end or at least reduction of cravings, not only for drugs or alcohol, but also for sugar. Energy levels also improved, as did sleeping problems if tryptophan was included in the amino acid formula. The new therapy dissolved the cocaine addicts' "wall." It was no longer an issue, and without that terrible discomfort, they could stay in treatment.

Kenneth Blum, Ph.D., a scientist specializing in the area of brain chemistry and addiction, explains addictive cravings as a largely genetic problem in the programming of the brain's mood chemistry via the neurotransmitters. More significantly, his research identified the missing piece in addiction recovery programs—amino acids.

Unfortunately, within a few years of Ross launching the amino acid therapy as part of the center's protocol, tryptophan was no longer available. (The Food and Drug Administration banned its use after people became ill from a contaminated batch of tryptophan.) After the ban of tryptophan, another blow prevented the use of amino acids from becoming standard practice in addiction treatment, as might have happened as news of the excellent results achieved with them reached treatment centers across the country. While some centers had begun using the amino acids for the treatment of substance abuse, the majority had not, and they were failing in an obvious way because of the crack cocaine epidemic.

"The relapse phenomenon wasn't a secret anymore," says Ross. "The insurance companies began to refuse to pay because the programs were obviously not working. You couldn't blame them. People were going back ten times for treatment, and each treatment cost at least $10,000, which in those days was the equivalent of $20,000 now." As insurance reimbursement dried up, residential treatment centers all over the United States went out of business.

The center where Ross worked was a privately funded nonprofit institution, one of the few in the country, so its doors remained open, and they were able to continue with the amino acid treatment with great success. In 1988, Ross established Recovery Systems, a clinic in Mill Valley, California, devoted to treating addiction, mood disorders, and eating disorders from a nutritional psychology orientation, with amino acids a central part of the protocol. Ross is currently director of the clinic and has detailed her method in two books, *The Mood Cure* and *The Diet Cure*.

Ross treats all kinds of addictions, with marijuana addiction, alcoholism, and addiction to stimulant drugs being the most common in her patient population. The first step in Ross's approach is to gather information about a client's full range of physical, emotional/psychological, and behavioral symptoms in an initial psychosocial assessment of that person and his or her family. A nutritional evaluation, medical workup, and specialized testing to determine vitamin and mineral status and blood sugar levels among other parameters are also part of the preliminaries to treatment.

Based on this information, Ross designs a treatment program for the individual that includes a supplement regimen, dietary recommendations, at least weekly consultation on nutrition, and some kind of ongoing peer support and individual, group, or family therapy several times a week, as needed. For those whose addiction is too entrenched to endeavor quitting on an outpatient basis, Ross recommends any of several residential programs that support the use of nutritional supplements and will tailor a diet according to Ross's specifications.

The amino acids (given in oral supplement form) are tailored to the individual's symptoms (see the following section). Standard features in the protocol are a multivitamin/mineral designed to balance blood sugar and vitamins B and C, especially during detox to help flush out toxins. "Vitamins B and C are probably the most badly needed. In fact, some addicts actually take B complex and C while they're using," notes Ross.

In general in cases of addiction, people need to take the amino acids for about a year. In some cases, although it is not common, people have only had to take them for three months. People can tell when they no longer need them because they no longer like them and their effects change, says Ross. "Something that used to be relaxing will make you tired; something that used to be stimulating will give you a headache. Once the amino acid has done the repair job, it doesn't have any benefits." For this reason, she encourages people after some months on an amino acid to try not taking it for a few days and see how they feel. If they don't miss it, she tells them to stay off it until they do. They may never need it again, but it's there in case they do, which is reassuring to many people.

 For more about amino acids, see chapter 2.

Identifying Amino Acid Deficiencies

In designing a treatment plan, it is necessary to identify the individual's neurotransmitter deficiencies, which underlie the negative mood states that emerge with the cessation of substance use. There is no direct test for determining the level of neurotransmitters in the brain, and while testing can identify the neurotransmitter and amino acid levels in the urine or blood, this is not a definitive indicator of brain levels, states Ross. Fortunately, the symptoms of deficiency of the neurotransmitters in question are "very obvious" and distinct from each other.

Symptoms of Neurotransmitter Deficiency or Dysfunction[196]

Serotonin

depression with negativity and
  anxiousness
low self-esteem
irritability, anger
anxiety, panic, phobias
obsessive thoughts/behaviors
suicidal ideation
sleep disturbances
heat intolerance
premenstrual syndrome

Dopamine/Norepinephrine

depression with apathy
lack of energy
lack of drive
focus and concentration
  problems

GABA

inability to relax
stressed-out or burned-out state
tight muscles

Endorphins

sensitivity to pain
emotional sensitivity
crying easily

Then the amino acid precursor of the deficient neurotransmitter can be given in supplement form to raise the levels of that neurotransmitter in the brain. By giving the body the amino acid building blocks for the neurotransmitters that are in short supply, "they can typically be replenished quickly, easily, and safely," Ross states.[194] If the person's diet has been chronically poor or other factors have resulted in overall amino acid depletion, a complete amino acid formula may also be indicated.[195]

As noted previously, depression and anxiety often go hand in hand with addiction. Both serotonin and dopamine/norepinephrine deficiencies are characterized by depression, but the depressions are of different kinds. With low serotonin, it is the anxious, agitated, restless, worried form of depression, the negative dark cloud variety, says Ross. "It is not the can't-get-out-of-bed kind. In fact, often they wish they could get *into* bed because they're up at night, sleepless, pacing, worrying, and having dark thoughts."

This cluster of symptoms may understandably cause people "to assume that they have perhaps been traumatized by early childhood or other distress," notes Ross, having heard this from numerous clients. This is not to say that trauma is not a contributing factor, but Ross has found that when these people take L-tryptophan or 5-HTP (5-hydroxy tryptophan; in the body, tryptophan is converted into 5-HTP and then into serotonin) to increase available serotonin, the symptoms disappear in most cases. For the majority of people, tryptophan and 5-HTP have identical effects; for a few people, one works better than the other. While 5-HTP is available over the counter, tryptophan can only be obtained through a doctor's prescription.

In contrast to that of serotonin, the depression manifested in dopamine/norepinephrine deficiency is not of the agitated variety. With this neurotransmitter deficiency, people "are tired, they can't concentrate, and their vitality and ambition are compromised," says Ross. L-tyrosine or L-phenylalanine is the amino acid supplement needed to reverse this deficiency.

A stressed-out, burned-out state is the number one symptom of GABA deficiency, says Ross. "People lacking in this neurotransmitter describe themselves as 'overwhelmed.' They're stiff; their posture tends to be stiff rather than relaxed." They are chronically in the fight-or-flight response, with its attendant adrenaline flow. GABA as an amino acid supplement is indicated in these cases. The other "relaxing aminos" taurine and glycine can be used as corollary calming agents, according to Ross.

Endorphin deficiency is also often a factor in addiction. When endorphins (see chapter 1) are low, the person has difficulty feeling pleasure and may seek substances to provide that sensation. Deficiency of endorphins, the natural painkillers, results in vulnerability to physical and emotional pain. Typical signs are being "overly sensitive to emotional injury. People hurt their feelings and they can't get over it," states Ross. "They're just emotionally exposed, raw." The amino acid building blocks for endorphins are DL-phenylalanine and D-phenylalanine.

L-glutamine is another amino acid that can be useful as general support and a source of fuel for the whole brain. Its primary role is to keep the blood sugar in the brain stable. The brain burns glutamine when it runs out of glucose in a hypoglycemic blood sugar drop, Ross explains. Supplementation with glutamine usually promotes "stable, calm, alert brain function."[197] It is typically needed when the person eats a lot of sweets and starches, has a high alcohol or caffeine intake, and skips meals.

The advantages of amino acid supplementation over prescription drugs aimed at neurotransmitter function (such as antianxiety and antidepressant drugs) to deal with the mood fallout of withdrawal from addiction are numerous. Unlike the drugs, which can take weeks to begin to work, supplementation produces effects rapidly, often in a matter of days, or even hours, says Ross. Also unlike drugs, amino acid supplementation addresses the underlying problems— that is, neurotransmitter deficiency and function—rather than manipulating brain chemistry in an unnatural way. Further, they eliminate other withdrawal symptoms as well as addictive cravings.

Julian: Marijuana and Sex Addiction

Julian was a very gifted classical musician and composer who had gotten a lot of recognition from a young age. He was successful, getting frequent commissions, and had married another musician with whom he was very much in love. Stress affected him greatly, however, and at 28, during a particularly difficult period when there was a lot of pressure on him to create, he began smoking marijuana. At the same time, he and his wife weren't having sex because, according to Julian, she had some sexual problems. He had been quite promiscuous before their marriage and began to look at pornography and masturbate, often several times a day, typically combined with smoking pot.

Only on pot did he feel that life was worth living. Marijuana gave him the illusion that life was exciting, that he was full of ideas, and that he could handle the stress at work and home. In actuality, it made the whole situation worse. Within six months of smoking almost every day, he found that he could not give it up, and over the next five years, his life "went entirely downhill."

Commissions came few and far between, he did less well with them, and he made less and less money. His relationship with his wife was nearing estrangement. Julian was smoking several times a day, unable to stop. His wife was very disturbed by this obvious addiction and pled with him to quit. He would try and sometimes was able to stay off it for a week, but always went back. Then he would lie to his wife about it, which he hated doing.

Along with the issue of addiction, his wife resented the money he spent on marijuana. He wasn't bringing in money because he couldn't get work, partly because he was unreliable and partly because his temperament had become so foul. He was depressed, irritable, paranoid, and not pleasant to be around. He suffered from insomnia and kept odd hours. He had no energy and was no longer motivated to pursue commissions or even to write music. He would have great ideas when he got high but then was unable to carry them out.

Julian didn't know whether it was that he was truly no longer interested in music or that he was so incapacitated by the marijuana he could no longer access his gift. He came to Ross to find out which it was, and because he couldn't stand lying to his wife. He was 33 by then and was well aware that his life had disintegrated before his eyes, the confidence of his earlier years gone. He suspected the pot had a lot to do with it. His inability to stop his obsessive masturbating had forced him to acknowledge that he had a sex addiction as well. He had tried to deal with his problems in psychotherapy, but it hadn't produced any change.

Julian had the classic symptoms of marijuana addiction—nonfunctioning, unmotivated, depressed, tired, irritable—which as mentioned previously is one of the most common addictions Ross treats. "This addiction often goes unrecognized because marijuana is not generally considered addictive."

As a drug, marijuana is insidious because it has the unique property among drugs of being fat-soluble, which means it gets stored in the brain, explains Ross. Alcohol, speed, cocaine, and heroin are all water-soluble, so they leave the brain and the body quickly. "This is why alcoholics often have remorse. The alcohol leaves their system quickly, so they intermittently have a chance to assess the damage, whereas a pothead is always high. They don't know it because they don't feel intoxicated, but they are still high. The majority of the brain is fatty tissue, so marijuana is stored there, affecting the brain and the personality." Ross notes that it generally takes six months to a year after quitting to get the pot out of the fat cells. Gradually, over months, "you begin to see what you are like free of the drug."

The first recommendation that Ross made to Julian was that he start going to Marijuana Anonymous. He refused, saying, "I'm so paranoid and depressed, I can't go anywhere. I'm certainly not going to sit with a bunch of people I don't know and talk about my addiction."

Ross made a deal with him then. He would follow the nutritional protocol and continue with his therapy. If this did not enable him to stop using, then he would need to go to Twelve-Step meetings or Ross would not be able to continue working with him because what they were doing would obviously not be enough. Julian agreed to this.

In Julian's case, a major dietary overhaul was not needed. He already ate healthfully. The only issues were that he was undereating and not getting much protein. He didn't have good muscle mass and wasn't able to exercise the way he did before. Ross recommended that he increase his caloric intake and eat fish and eggs to get more protein. Though he was a vegetarian, he was willing to eat these foods.

To improve his energy, one of Ross's staff nutritionists gave him the amino acid tyrosine. To help him cope better with stress, he took GABA, B vitamins, and vitamin C. GABA would help improve his sleep as well, for which he also took 5-HTP and melatonin (a hormone produced by the pineal gland that regulates the sleep-wake cycle). Saliva testing had revealed that he was only slightly above the stage of profound adrenal exhaustion (breakdown of the adrenal system and its ability to respond to stress). The GABA, B complex, and vitamin C would all help with this, and his nutritionist started him on a short-term course of the adrenal hormones DHEA (dehydroepiandrosterone) and pregnenolone along with the herb licorice as further adrenal support.

Most important to ending his addictions, however, was DL-phenylalanine to correct his low endorphin levels, which were indicated by the primary purpose of the pot being to provide pleasure. "He really didn't experience any pleasure in his life except what the pot gave him," says Ross.

"The DL-phenylalanine had an almost immediate impact on the marijuana smoking," Ross recalls. Within 24 hours, he had stopped smoking, and it was no struggle for him to maintain that. The masturbation continued for another couple of months, but not nearly as frequently. Instead of several times a day, it went down to a couple of times a week.

Of his sex addiction, Ross comments, "When your endorphins are low and you have no capacity to feel pleasure, you have to go to extremes sometimes to get any pleasure. Sex was the only thing besides pot that briefly made him feel good. For somebody else, an ice cream sundae would do it, but with him, it had to be masturbation. When he built up his capacity to feel pleasure just from watching a sunset or taking walks, he was fine." His sexual appetite lost the obsessive component and became normal.

In some cases of addiction, "correcting the brain chemistry is enough," states Ross. It was not necessary for Julian to go the one step further in treatment by attending Marijuana Anonymous. Nor did he need to make major life changes. He had a sober wife, smoked in private, and did not have a lot of pothead friends. He needed only to return to the good life that was already in place and to the person he was meant to be.

Once his wife could see that the nightmare was over, that he had stopped smoking, which the change in him made obvious, she opened up more. They went to counseling together, and their sex life became more satisfying.

Julian got his answer about whether music still had meaning for him. Off marijuana, his interest, energy, motivation, and ambition all returned. "It all came back to him pretty quickly," says Ross.

At six weeks after starting on the nutritional program, Julian reported that his work output had greatly increased, he had stretches of excitement again that were not induced by pot, and his sleep rhythm was getting back to normal. He was going to bed at 11 P.M. and getting up at 7 A.M., something he hadn't done in years. His stress level was lower, and his mood had lifted. At that point, his nutritionist had him stop taking the DHEA, pregnenolone, and licorice.

Five months into treatment, his work output was back to where it had been before his life began disintegrating, and he was getting commissions again. He was still taking DL-phenylalanine, tyrosine, and the vitamins, but using 5-HTP, melatonin, and GABA only as needed.

Julian consulted with Ross periodically for a year. It has now been two years since he has seen her. He recently wrote to say that he is still off marijuana and only rarely needs to use the amino acids. He expressed his gratitude and reported that he and his wife are very happy and his career is going beautifully.

Neurotransmitter Restoration: Intravenous Amino Acids

The William Hitt Center in Tijuana, Mexico, uses a protocol based on the same principles as those operational in Julia Ross's approach to addiction, except the amino acids, along with requisite vitamins and minerals, are delivered intravenously during a ten-day residential treatment program. The protocol, termed Neurotransmitter Restoration (NTR), was developed by William M. Hitt, Doctor of Medicine and Surgery (a Mexican medical credential) and an international member of both the Canadian Psychiatric Association and the American Psychiatric Association. He also holds a doctorate in applied biology and is a researcher in immunocytopharmacology (the study of the effects of substances on immune cells and immunity). Over the last 20 years, Dr. Hitt has used NTR to treat over 6,000 people with addictions.

"The success rate of our treatment is around 95 percent among the people who deal with the psychological and spiritual aspects of addiction," states Dr. Hitt. By this he means that Neurotransmitter Restoration can successfully get a person off drugs or alcohol, but it is up to the individual to make the necessary changes in his or her life to support not using.

"The success rate of our treatment is around 95 percent among the people who deal with the psychological and spiritual aspects of addiction," states Dr. Hitt. By this he means that NTR can redress neurotransmitter deficiencies and imbalances and, in so doing, remove cravings and prevent withdrawal symptoms, which successfully gets a person off drugs or alcohol, but it is up to the individual to make the necessary changes in his or her life to support not using.

"No one who leaves this program after ten days has any craving for the drug that they came in using. If you knock out the craving, you're 50 percent of the way. Now you have to link into a support group that can help you along because life is not just ten days, or 30 days, or however long a treatment program is."

Yes, ten days of intravenous amino acids are sufficient to correct the imbalance of neurotransmitters in the brain. In fact, says Dr. Hitt, eight days would be sufficient in most cases, but he uses ten in his program to ensure that rebalance is indeed complete. Occasionally, he has had to keep patients for 12 or 13 days. In these cases, the patients neglected to tell Dr. Hitt about one of their addictions and only did so when some of the brain fog of addiction lifted after the first week of detoxification. They then needed additional treatment to address a different set of neurotransmitters. All patients are given oral supplements of amino acids as stabilizers to take at home, but the work of rebalancing has already been accomplished.

Not only can the neurotransmitters typically be rebalanced in ten days, but the brain retains the balance, unless the person does something to cause an imbalance again, says Dr. Hitt. "That is why the social aspect, or the psychological aspect, becomes very important. If you put the person back into the same zoo, he is probably going to use again. If they go back to using, and get their brain chemistry off again, their craving is just going to increase."

With amino acids, as all clinicians who use them know, the horrendous withdrawal symptoms associated with detoxing at a conventional rehabilitation center can be avoided. "That's the thing that most heroin addicts fear," observes Dr. Hitt. "They want to get off the heroin, but they're afraid to get off it because of the withdrawal. In this program, there's almost no withdrawal." Some people may sweat a little for a few hours, feel slightly nauseous, or have a little diarrhea, but none of it is terribly uncomfortable or clinically significant. "We've never had a heavy clinical withdrawal in 6,000 patients." In addition to amino acids and vitamins, the IV treatment during detoxification includes extra magnesium and potassium to replace the electrolytes (salts of sodium, potassium, and magnesium and other substances in the blood, tissue fluids, and cells that conduct an electrical charge) being depleted during the energy output of the withdrawal process, an important component in preventing withdrawal symptoms.

Most of the people who come to the Hitt Center have multiple addictions, such as to heroin and cocaine, or cocaine and alcohol along with five or six prescription drugs from their doctor. Iatrogenic (physician-induced) addictions are common. For a while, Dr. Hitt was getting a lot of patients who had gone into other centers for alcohol treatment and come out addicted to Valium. The current trend seems to be people who have become addicted to prescription drugs they obtained over the internet, including Vicodin and methadone.

Crystal methamphetamine is an exception to the multiple addiction norm because the drug is so very satisfying to those who are addicted to it, says Dr. Hitt. "What you'll hear from them is something like this: Their idea of ecstasy would be to have a mound of crystal, to be on an island by themselves with a Bible, and just sitting there, free to use as much crystal as they wanted."

Crystal meth is not the most addictive of the substances people use, however. "The two most addictive substances I deal with in treatment are nicotine and crack cocaine," says Dr. Hitt. He places the addictive profile (how addictive a substance is) for these two substances at 99 percent, while heroin and alcohol are at 60 percent; crystal methamphetamine at 55 to 60 percent; cocaine at 48; and marijuana at 17.

While crack cocaine and nicotine are the most addictive substances, diazepam or Valium-like drugs are the most dangerous to withdraw from, says Dr. Hitt. There is a high risk of seizure, so "you have to go very slowly." In addition, these drugs, unlike the others (aside from marijuana, as noted earlier), are stored in fat cells, so will still be in the body for months after the initial detoxification. For those who are overweight, the time it takes for the drug to be out of the body is even longer.

Addiction and Dopamine

"Most people that have addiction problems are born with a deficiency of dopamine," states Dr. Hitt. "This is true with any obsessive-compulsive behavior. Substance abuse is one form of obsessive-compulsive behavior." Addiction to chemicals, sex, gambling, food, or work all have their root in dopamine. The substances or activities are dopaminergic, meaning they affect dopamine activity in the brain. Addictive use is an attempt to correct dopamine deficiency, and cravings arise from the imbalance, he explains.

While other neurotransmitters may be involved, dopamine must always be addressed in treatment, according to Dr. Hitt. For example, while dopamine is the neurotransmitter to address in addiction to alcohol, Valium, marijuana, glue (as in glue-sniffing), or nicotine, serotonin and endorphins must be addressed along with dopamine in cases of addiction to crack cocaine, crystal, and heroin. "No matter what drugs you're treating or what neurotransmitters you're working on, you always have to end up working with dopamine," Dr. Hitt concludes. "That is the genetic basis of all addictions. If dopamine is thrown off, then it can throw some of the other neurotransmitters off."

This raises an important point regarding cigarette smoking, which is common among former alcoholics and drug addicts. If the neurotransmitters were not rebalanced during their detoxification from drugs or alcohol, it is understandable why they smoke—once again, it is an attempt to rebalance the dopamine. If the neurotransmitters were rebalanced during detoxification, as at the Hitt Center, then smoking afterward is likely to throw the neurotransmitters out of balance again. "If they're smoking after they detox, they're more likely to relapse because they're exacerbating the dopamine problem again," notes Dr. Hitt. "You've got to look at nicotine as a powerful drug."

Dr. Hitt has dedicated his life to bringing awareness of the amino acid solution to the field of addiction treatment. "If you could see the people coming out of here, you would say, 'Anyone who would not do this would have to be completely out of their mind.' But you've got to realize that most things in medicine are very slow. You have to be patient and willing to take it on the chin a bit if you're changing a discourse, but I won't be content until the world has an opportunity to at least know about this, so at least people can have the opportunity to get free of drugs."

The following cases illustrate the range and severity of the addictions that Dr. Hitt has successfully treated at his center.

In Their Own Words

"Over the next 15 years I manipulated doctors, dentists, therapists, emergency room personnel, pharmaceutical drug representatives, and friends to get an array of different pills. Topping my list of choice pills were Librium, Darvon, Elavil, Demerol, Haldol, Halcion, Tranxene, Darvocet, Percocet, Percodan, Flexeril, Xanax, and Ativan, to name a few."

—Cindy R. Mogil, author of *Swallowing a Bitter Pill*[198]

From Prescription Drugs to Crack

A woman, 42, was addicted to 15 prescription drugs, including Prozac, the painkiller Dilaudid, Valium and other tranquilizers, and methadone. She had requested the latter from a doctor to ease the pain of shingles. Despite the drugs, she complained of constant pain. She also had drug-induced psychosis with paranoia. She had been on multiple prescriptions for about ten years, but her use had become more chronic in the past two years.

When her mother brought her to Dr. Hitt in desperation, she weighed a mere 68 pounds (she was 5 feet, one inch in height). She ate little and had constant diarrhea, to the point that she had to wear adult diapers. She was unable to do anything in her life, including care for herself or her home.

At the end of the ten days of treatment at the Hitt Center, she was off all her medications, and her weight had gone up to 84 pounds because the diarrhea was resolved, she was eating again, and she was now able to absorb the nutrients from what she ate. She no longer complained of pain. Parenthetically, Dr. Hitt had seen no evidence of shingles and believes that her pain was psychological in origin. "Chronic pain medication often begets more pain," he notes.

As she was still in such a weak condition after the initial ten days, she was one of the people that Dr. Hitt treated for longer. "Her

75

immune system was completely shot. I brought her back as an immunological patient so I could monitor her weekly." She came for an appointment every week (later she cut down to monthly) and received further intravenous amino acids, vitamins, and minerals to build up her system slowly. Over the course of her treatment, she received all four of the formulas that Dr. Hitt uses in Neurotransmitter Restoration.

Within a couple of months, she became functional enough to start going to church with her mother and sister again, as she used to before she became so ill. Her drug-induced psychosis was gone. Over six months, her weight got up to 125 pounds. It has now been four years since her treatment. She has not returned to using drugs in that time, and she is now able to work and support herself.

A 35-year-old stockbroker with a wife and new baby was doing 75 Vicodin a day. His habit had built up over a period of six to seven years. He bought the drug illicitly and would stay high all the time. After ten days of treatment, he went home, minus his habit, and has been fine ever since.

A CEO of a company, 34, looked like he was doing everything right. He was rich and successful, with a lovely wife and a beautiful home. People noticed that he was hyper but concluded that most CEOs are and didn't think anything was amiss. He had been using for ten years and had tried different programs to quit, but nothing had worked. One night, he forgot that he and his wife were having a dinner party for 30 people. He was off doing cocaine somewhere and didn't come home. His wife covered for him, saying that he was ill. After that, he knew he had to do something and checked into the Hitt Center. He's been well for almost a year and a half now.

A 31-year-old man came to Dr. Hitt for treatment of his crack cocaine addiction. He had an alcoholic father, with whom he ran a business. "When he went into the crack addiction, which usually also takes people into a sex addiction, his behavior patterns started changing immensely," recalls Dr. Hitt. His work and home life fell apart. His wife divorced him and took the kids. But he didn't hit rock-bottom until he tried to sell his body to get money for drugs. Whether he sold his body to a man or woman didn't matter to him; all he cared about was getting the money. He told Dr. Hitt that he gave up because "nobody would buy me." It was at this point that he sought treatment, which was successful.

Seeing the results, the man's father, then 57, decided to get treatment for his alcoholism. He had been drinking for 40 years. The father was flying from the East Coast to Los Angeles, where a friend was to meet his plane and drive him down to the Hitt Center in Tijuana. The friend called the center, saying that the man had not been on the plane. It turns out that he had sexually harassed a flight attendant and been escorted off the plane at a stopover in Atlanta. The airlines rerouted him. When he finally arrived in Los Angeles, the only way the friend could get him to the clinic was to offer him a bottle of vodka. "He had started out to come to the clinic of his own volition, but by the time he got here, that vodka looked pretty good to him," recalls Dr. Hitt. "He came in drunk."

But that was the last time he had a drink. Father and son have been "clean" for five years and are back to work.

In the following account, one of Dr. Hitt's patients tells about her serious, long-term addiction to crystal methamphetamine and how she was able to overcome it through his Neurotransmitter Restoration program.

In Their Own Words:
Celeste on Crystal Meth Addiction

I was 23; I had finished with college and had a master's degree in psychology. My boyfriend at the time offered me a line of crystal. I willingly tried it. It felt like the best thing that had happened to me for years. I didn't need to eat; I had plenty of energy to do everything that I wanted to do; I felt happy and clear-headed, and it was wonderful.

I come from a good upper-middle-class family that put me through college. I had a typical 1980s college experience. I smoked plenty of pot and drank alcohol, but that honestly never hindered me from doing anything that I felt I should do. I wrote papers after doing a bong. I would get drunk on the weekends but then not drink all week. Alcohol and pot never seemed like a problem for me at all. If I ran out of pot, it was fine.

As soon as I tried meth, I started seeking it out. I don't think I became addicted right away, even though I loved it. After probably six months to a year of weekend use, I realized that I was somewhat addicted to it. I began spending more money on it and using it more often. Around that time, I got a job working in a mental health facility with teenagers who had behavioral problems, which was really ironic. Some of the kids there were using drugs. I tried not to work on the substance abuse unit because I would have felt like a hypocrite.

I didn't have a huge crowd of people around me who were using drugs. It was mostly just my boyfriend and one or two friends of his. I was careful to hide my addiction; that is, if I would do a line in the morning before I went to work, I would check my nose and put on perfume because the crystal had a certain odor. I put all kinds of energy into hiding what I was doing, and I was pretty good at it because I never did get in any trouble at work.

I just felt horrible about myself for using, for one thing, because I knew that I was addicted, and I hated it. But I felt worse not using at all, because I would be tired and depressed, angry, and just completely uncomfortable. So I continued to seek it out. I ended up through my addiction, marrying a crystal dealer, who I met through the boyfriend who gave me my first line. I threw away an opportunity to go into the Peace Corps in order to be near him while he was in jail—this was before we were married.

I was able to hide my addiction from my family. I told them my boyfriend was in jail for marijuana. My dad said, "What kind of people are you hanging around with? What are you doing?" I was able to rationalize it. I also got into church and spirituality while I was using, so I was able to rationalize it that way. "He's a good person in his heart, and it doesn't matter," was what I said.

My family could have disowned me and I still would have been with him and I still would have kept on using. But I was miserable the whole time that I was with him. I was miserable that I was using, but I couldn't stop, and it was convenient because I had his house to live in. Even though he was in prison, he still had plenty of drugs. He was in prison when I married him. That's embarrassing and that's sick.

My family didn't know the whole story, but they knew that I married him in jail. They asked me, "What are you doing?" They still didn't know that I was using drugs; they just knew that I wasn't very interested in working, that I was underemployed—by that I mean, with a master's degree, I was earning nine and ten dollars an hour.

By then I'd gone on to another job, in social work. But I wasn't really digging into a career. I felt like I was just spinning my wheels, and painting the walls in his house, working in the garden, and just doing the things that I wanted, but I wasn't moving ahead with my life. I looked like a functioning member of society, but I was very skinny and pale. I hate to look at pictures of myself from that time.

When I was on crystal in the beginning, it did make me feel up and happy, talkative and social. But as I got more into using, I began to be withdrawn and nervous. I would start to get stir crazy in the house, but I wouldn't want to go out until after it was dark because I would feel uncomfortable talking to somebody. I would go to the grocery store, and having to hand my money to the clerk made me anxious because I was worried my hand would shake.

After my husband got out of jail, I was pregnant within the first two months. I was actually able to stop using all during my pregnancy. Whether it was a hormonal surge or I just knew that that was something you didn't do, I thought, "Oh, thank God, I got pregnant, because this baby saved my life, how wonderful."

Then within probably four months after my son was born, while I was still breast-feeding, I began using again. That's something I feel awful about. I was just going to use one more time to get all the laundry done and clean the house and so forth, and it became stronger and stronger. I was different in a lot of ways from most addicts in that I was able to maintain work somewhat, my son was never taken away from me, and he was never hungry. But still, I was driving 40 miles to pick up the substance and 40 miles back, and then two days later the same thing.

My father died during this time and left me a large inheritance. I blew a lot of it on drugs, but thank God I had the wherewithal and made it to Dr. Hitt.

I may not have gone into that huge downward spiral to living on the streets, but, believe me, I was just as addicted as the person on the street. I had tried everything to quit. I tried church, I tried fundamental Christianity, I tried hypnosis, past-life regression. I went to NA [Narcotics Anonymous] meetings, I went to AA meetings. I prayed and I prayed and I prayed. I did affirmations. I did psychology; I read every book on addiction that I could find. I think that if it had been purely a psychological or an emotional thing, through all the things that I did, I would have been able to quit.

One day [she was 33 by this time] I was reading this kind of back-street spiritual publication, and there was a very small ad that said, "Freedom from drugs, no withdrawals, no cravings, 10-day outpatient program." And I went, "Oh, my God, that can't be real. I would know about it," because I was working in a hospital at the time. I was into psychology. Like NA and AA say, there are no magical solutions. But I was desperate for one. So I called and got down to the clinic.

Dr. Hitt is so wise and so humble and so sincere and brilliant. Everything he told me made so much sense. I felt like it was something in my brain I had no control over. There was still a part in my mind that thought, "Well, if this was true, everybody would know about it." But the next day I started treatment. I was ready. I did a big line before I went in, and they cleared it all out.

Dr. Hitt put me on the IV. From the first treatment, I felt a huge difference. I felt like I didn't have that itch where I was just waiting for the opportunity to go do another line. Even though I was tired during the treatment, I wasn't angry, I wasn't wolfing chocolates like I would do usually when I was coming down. There was no irritability. I just felt like I needed to take a nap.

The treatment was ten days, and then it tapered off. I know he's changed it since I went through it. After the ten days, I felt completely free of it. I didn't go to NA and AA meetings, but I was in karate and moving up through the different belts at the time, so I did have another outlet and something that I was focused on. I think everybody needs something besides just the treatment, some sort of a goal, a support group—NA or AA is fine. But his treatment just made it so easy for me to focus on the better things in my life and focus on getting better. Before, I felt like I couldn't.

I had no cravings at all. There have been times in my life since then where I've felt low and I thought, gosh, it would be nice to have the energy to go ahead and paint the walls or whatever, and maybe if somebody had come to my front door with it, I might have used it. But that just hasn't happened. Like I say, it wasn't in my social circle.

Six months after I went through treatment, I pooled the rest of the money my dad had given me in his inheritance and bought a house. I got into a teaching program, which took about a year and a half. Now [at 38] I'm in my third year of teaching. I teach second grade.

My husband and I got a divorce. My son is nine years old now, and he's fine and healthy, but I do watch him and I am concerned about him because he comes from two parents with a propensity towards crystal. I'm going to be very careful, believe me, when he gets into his teens and has a possibility of being exposed to that kind of thing.

This treatment works. I think that when everything in your brain is so out of whack, it's impossible to quit drugs no matter how much you want to. It's such a struggle. In the NA and AA meetings—I know they work for some people and God bless them for that—it's just everybody saying, "My name is so-and-so and I'm an addict." I didn't want to classify myself as that. I didn't want to keep on reinforcing that. I wanted to not be an addict anymore, and I feel like Dr. Hitt's treatment did that for me.

My desire to quit when I tried all those other ways was very high. I went to Kaiser, and they told me you're going to need to go to meetings, you're going to need to go to education classes about drugs. I already knew about drugs. I could teach about drugs. I just knew that wasn't going to do it, because I still really wanted it, even though I hated myself for wanting it.

My message to other addicts is: Be willing to try NTR. Be open to it. It is very real. If a person is ready to quit, this makes it very easy. But you have to have drives and goals beyond that, too. I believe there has to be a reason why you want to quit.

4 *Allergies and Addiction*: NAET

When most people think of allergies, they think of reactions that cause you to stay away from the problem foods or substances. In actuality, you may crave the very thing to which you are allergic.

"An allergy can manifest as an addiction or an aversion," explains allergy authority Devi S. Nambudripad, M.D., D.C., L.Ac., Ph.D., of Buena Park, California. "It can go either way. I treat people with addiction for allergies because they're allergic to something that is causing them to be addicted to the substance."

Dr. Nambudripad's work has transformed the field of allergy treatment. In the early 1980s, she developed a highly effective, noninvasive, painless method of both identifying and eliminating allergies—NAET (Nambudripad's Allergy Elimination Techniques)—which is now practiced worldwide by over 7,000 healthcare practitioners. Dr. Nambudripad and other NAET practitioners have found that with the elimination of allergies, people easily and naturally lose their addictions.

According to Dr. Nambudripad, allergies are "energy incompatibilities" that create energy blockages in the body. That is, the body's energy field regards the energy field of a substance—inhaled, ingested, or otherwise contacted—as incompatible with its own, and its presence disturbs the flow of energy along the body's meridians (the energy channels as described in acupuncture). One, several, or even all the meridians may be affected. The central nervous system records the energy disturbance and is then programmed to regard the substance as toxic. NAET uses chiropractic and acupuncture techniques to restore the smooth flow of energy along the meridians and reprogram the central nervous system no longer to regard the substance as incompatible energetically.

Dr. Nambudripad has found that people with addiction are most often allergic to the drug or other substance to which they are addicted. Further, in every one of the hundreds of cases of addiction (whether to food, drugs, alcohol, tobacco, caffeine, or other substance) that Dr. Nambudripad has treated to date, the person was allergic to B vitamins and sugar.

"B complex is a nerve food," she explains. "B vitamins are necessary for all the enzymatic functions of the body. With an allergy to the B complex, you cannot absorb these vitamins properly. If you are not absorbing them, your body craves them." Sugar is closely related to the B vitamins, "which cannot be absorbed on their own. They are large molecules and need to be connected or hooked to the glucose (sugar) molecules." What happens with a sugar allergy is that "you cannot digest or assimilate the complex carbohydrates,"[199] which contain B vitamins. The result is sugar craving as a quick source of the energy that glucose provides the body.

> **Dr. Nambudripad has found that people with addiction are most often allergic to the drug or other substance to which they are addicted. Further, in every one of the hundreds of cases of addiction (whether to food, drugs, alcohol, tobacco, caffeine, or other substance) that Dr. Nambudripad has treated to date, the person was allergic to B vitamins and sugar.**

Thus, allergies to B vitamins and sugar explain the carbohydrate and sugar cravings that underlie addiction. In addition to these cravings, the body may also seek substances and activities that compensate for the deficient nutrients, such as alcohol. "A small amount of alcohol can satisfy the body's immediate need for sugar, temporarily. This is the reason most people feel a surge of energy or well-being soon after they take a few sips of alcohol. But the sense of well-being does not last long."[200] The feeling of well-being, which comes from giving the brain the fuel it

In Their Own Words

"I once heard a woman say that as an alcoholic, a part of her will always be deeply attracted to alcohol. . . . The attraction—the pull, the hunger, the yearning—doesn't die when you say good-bye to the drink."

—Caroline Knapp, author of *Drinking: A Love Story*, on her alcoholism[201]

needs, is the driving force behind the addiction.

Ending cravings by eliminating allergies happens in two ways. First, eliminating allergies to nutrients opens the way for proper nutritive absorption, which in turn corrects the deficiencies and ends cravings for compensating substances. Second, removing allergies to the addictive substances themselves removes the craving for those substances.

Allergy elimination is beneficial to the health in other ways. It improves digestion, lifts a large burden from the immune system, and reduces the toxic load on the liver, which enables it to better perform its function of detoxifying the body—a vital role given the toxins that accumulate as a result of addiction to drugs or other harmful substances.

Along with eliminating the allergies, Dr. Nambudripad treats addiction with large doses of B-complex vitamin supplements (300 to 500 mg daily of a combination formula) to replenish the deficient nutrients more quickly than can happen through diet. This supplementation further helps to reduce the cravings for the addictive substance, which is especially important during the withdrawal period.

The effects of the allergies extend far beyond cravings, however. For example, "[m]any people who go through Alcoholics Anonymous and similar groups will learn to quit drinking by practicing self-control, group therapy, support systems, etc.," observes Dr. Nambudripad. "But most of them end up having some physical pain: migraines, headaches, neck pains, shoulder pains, insomnia, etc. When they are treated for B complex, sugar, and alcohol, their physical symptoms disappear."[202]

About NAET

NAET uses kinesiology's muscle response testing (MRT) to identify allergies. Chiropractic and acupuncture techniques are then

Symptoms of Allergies

The following are some of the many symptoms and conditions associated with allergies.[203] You can see that they range far beyond the runny nose and teary eyes most often thought of in connection to allergies. Note that anxiety, carbohydrate cravings, and obsessive-compulsive disorder are all associated with addiction (see chapters 3 and 8).

anxiety

attention deficit

Candida/yeast overgrowth

chronic fatigue

craving for
    carbohydrates/chocolate

distractibility

eczema

frequent colds, bronchial infections, and other infections

headaches

hypoglycemia

hyperactivity

impulsivity

indigestion

insomnia

irritable bowel syndrome

leaky gut syndrome

mood swings

nervous stomach

obsessive-compulsive disorder

phobias

poor appetite

poor memory

restless leg syndrome

sinusitis

toxicity (reactivity/sensitivity) to
    mercury and other heavy
    metals

implemented to remove the energy blockages in the body that underlie allergies and to reprogram the brain and nervous system not to respond allergically to previously problem substances.

Like many revolutionary inventions, NAET began with an accidental discovery. Dr. Nambudripad, who had long been allergic to nearly everything, one day ate some carrot while she was cooking the two foods she could safely eat—white rice and broccoli. Within moments of eating the carrot, she "felt like [she] was going to pass out."[204] She used muscle response testing to check for an allergy to carrots and was not surprised that she tested highly allergic.

A student of acupuncture at the time, she gave herself an acupuncture treatment, with the help of her husband, to keep from going into shock. She fell asleep with the needles still inserted in specific acupuncture

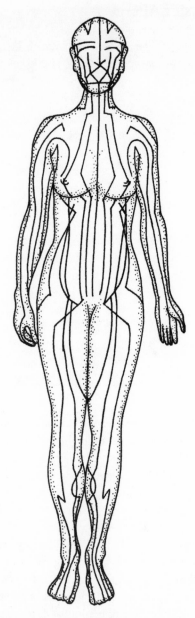

Acupuncture Meridians

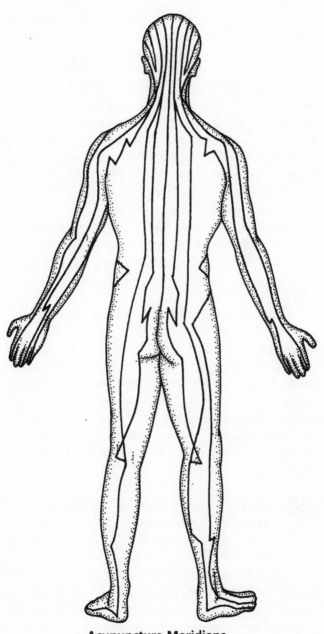

Acupuncture Meridians

points, and when she woke almost an hour later, she no longer felt sick and tired. In her hand were pieces of the carrot she had been eating. When she repeated the MRT, she no longer tested allergic to carrots. To check the validity of this result, she ate some carrot—no reaction.[205]

Dr. Nambudripad then ate bits of other foods to which she knew she was allergic and her reactions were as they had been—she was still allergic. "[S]o I knew my assumption was correct. My allergy to carrot was gone because of my contact with the carrot while undergoing acupuncture. My energy and the carrot's energy were repelling prior to the acupuncture treatment. After the treatment, their energies became similar—no more repulsion!"[206] She then tried this technique, which she later named NAET, on other foods to which she was allergic. The same thing happened—the allergies disappeared. After many years of living with pervasive allergies, she was able to systematically eliminate them and restore her health.

How NAET Works

NAET is based on the medical model of acupuncture, in which disease is diagnosed and treated as an energy imbalance in one or more of the body's meridians, or energy pathways. These meridians—there are 12 major ones—carry the body's vital energy, or *qi (chi),* to organs and throughout the system. Acupuncturists rebalance a meridian's energy by treating acupoints, the points on the body's surface that correspond to that meridian. Via the painless and very shallow insertion of needles or the application of pressure, the acupuncturist can remove energy blockages, get stagnant energy moving, or calm an overactive energy meridian.

 For more about acupuncture, see chapter 5. For more about NAET, see chapter 7.

Muscle Response Testing

The energy disturbance created by an allergy is the key to muscle response testing. To be tested for a potential allergen (something that causes an allergic reaction), you hold a vial containing the substance in one hand. You hold your other arm straight out in front of you and attempt to keep it there while the person testing pushes lightly down on it. Normally, you can easily hold your arm in place, but when you are allergic to the substance in the vial, your muscle response is weakened by the energy disturbance the allergy causes. A weakened response in testing indicates a possible allergy.

Those who have not experienced this test often find it difficult to believe that it can tell you anything, much less identify allergies. Upon undergoing the test, however, most people are amazed to discover that their arm seems to have a life, or mind, of its own. One moment, while holding one test substance, they see their arm drop slightly, and the next, with a different test vial, the arm holds steady. The person being tested usually does not know what's in the vial, so that does not influence the outcome.

For the treatment phase, the person holds the vial of the offending substance while the NAET practitioner uses slight pressure, needles, or a chiropractic tool to treat the appropriate points to clear the affected meridian(s). Keeping the vial in your energy field during this process reprograms the brain and nervous system to regard the substance as innocuous. In general, it is then necessary to avoid ingesting or otherwise having contact with the substance for 25 hours after treatment.

Dr. Nambudripad explains the reason for this time period: "An energy molecule takes 24 hours to travel through the body completing its circulation through all 12 major meridians, their branches, and sub-branches. It takes two hours to travel through one meridian. . . . When the allergy is treated through NAET, the patient has to wait 24 hours to let the energy molecule carrying the new information pass through the complete cycle of the journey."[207]

To be safe, one hour is added to the 24-hour cycle. If the person eats the allergenic food or has contact with an allergenic substance before the cycle is complete, the clearing treatment will likely have to be repeated and the food or other substance will need to be avoided for another 25 hours.

Common Allergens

While you can have sensitivities or allergies to anything you eat, drink, inhale, or touch or are touched by, such as fabric, cosmetics, chemicals, and environmental pollutants, many people share allergies to the same basic substances.

For the purposes of clearing people of their allergies more quickly, NAET combines the most common allergens in five basic groups: egg mix (egg white, egg yolk, chicken, and the antibiotic tetracycline, which is routinely fed to chickens to prevent infections); calcium mix (breast milk, cow's milk, goat's milk, milk albumin, casein, lactic acid, calcium, and coumarin, a phenolic or natural component found in milk); vitamin C (fruits, vegetables, vinegar, citrus, and berry); B-complex vitamins (17 vitamins in the B family); and sugar mix (cane, corn, maple, grape, rice, brown, and beet sugars, plus molasses, honey, fructose, dextrose, glucose, and maltose).

As noted earlier, in Dr. Nambudripad's clinical experience, allergies to the B-complex vitamins and sugar are universal among people with addictions.

For some people, it is sufficient to clear the five basic groups, but people with chronic addictions may have more extensive allergies. The larger basic collection of allergens includes magnesium, essential fatty acid oils, amino acids, grain mix (including gluten, the protein in grains), yeast mix (including acidophilus), artificial sweeteners, food additives, and food coloring, among others.

Artificial sweeteners, food additives, and food coloring contain chemicals that are neurotoxic to some individuals. NAET practitioners would say that the neurotoxicity stems from the fact that the individuals are allergic to the substances. Once cleared of the allergy, in most cases, people can eat foods containing these additives without suffering the negative effects, but it is a good idea for general health reasons to avoid these chemicals. Clearing allergies to gluten and casein (the protein in dairy products, included in the NAET calcium mix) can also enable people to eat formerly problematic foods, which is good news for those who have struggled with a gluten-free and/or casein-free diet.

It is worthwhile to note at this point that people can develop allergies to anything, even to nutrients that are natural to and required by the body. Says Dr. Nambudripad, "Any substance under the sun, including sunlight itself, can cause an allergic reaction in any individual."[208] The body can even develop a reactivity to its own tissue and brain chemicals, such as an allergy to one's own brain, hypothalamus, nerves, lung tissue, and neurotransmitters such as serotonin.

A Word about Gluten

Gluten is a protein found in wheat, barley, rye, oats, and other cereal grains and added to many commercial foods. During digestion, this large protein (consisting of long chains of amino acids) is first broken down into smaller peptides before being further reduced into its amino acid components. Peptides are similar to endorphins, substances that athletes know as the source of "runner's high." The peptide form of gluten is called glutemorphin. It is an opioid, meaning that it has an opium-like effect on brain cells.[209]

Gluten is difficult to digest, and many people develop an intolerance to it, which means that the body regards it as a foreign substance and the immune system launches an immune reaction against it. In addition, researchers theorize that incomplete digestion of gluten leads to excessive absorption of glutemorphins from the intestines into the bloodstream, which leads in turn to their passage across the blood-brain barrier where they exert their opioid effects.[210] In so doing, they depress serotonin, dopamine, and norepinephrine levels in the brain.[211] The opioid aspect also leads people to become addicted to gluten products.

While the intake of carbohydrates in general initially increases serotonin levels, chronic intake dramatically reduces serotonin levels in the brain. Typical results are a craving for carbohydrates, depression, sleep problems, and irritability.[212]

Eating foods that prompt an immune system reaction (foods to which one is sensitive or allergic) can actually interfere with neurotransmitter function. In regard to gluten, research has found that when people who are sensitive to gluten eat food containing it, their neurological function is altered.[213]

The Nature of Allergies

Allergic reactions tend to affect certain organs or meridians in individuals, depending on where their weak or vulnerable areas are, says Dr. Nambudripad. The organ most affected is known as the "target organ." The weakness can be genetic in nature or created by environmental factors such as toxic exposure or lack of adequate nutrition. The target organ can be the nervous system or the brain. If that is the case, chronic allergic reaction can negatively affect brain and nervous system function. In the case of food allergies, "with the first bite of an allergic food, the brain begins to block the energy channels, attempting to prevent the adverse energy of the food from entering into the body," says Dr. Nambudripad.[214]

As for how the allergies or sensitivities develop in the first place, Dr. Nambudripad cites heredity, toxins, weakened immunity, emotional stress, overexposure to a substance, and radiation. Anything that causes energy blockages in the body, which throws off the body's electromagnetic field, can cause an allergy to develop, she says. Toxins of any kind, from the neurotoxin mercury to the by-products of bacterial infection, disturb energy flow, as do synthetic food additives and artificial sweeteners.

The electromagnetic fields (EMFs) of televisions, computers, and other electrical devices in the house are a common culprit in the development of allergies, according to Dr. Nambudripad. The practice of feeding infants and children in front of the television so they will keep quiet and cooperate can be a recipe for allergies. The television's EMF extends at least 20 feet, she notes, and throws off the child's own energy field.

You could say that it "short-circuits the energy patterns," she says. And it does so while the child is eating, which is akin to doing NAET in reverse, programming the child to be allergic to that food. NAET removes the energy blockages underlying allergies, which returns the individual's electromagnetic field to its normal state.

The following three cases demonstrate how long-term addiction can be resolved with the NAET approach.

Estelle: End of a Lifetime Smoking Addiction

Estelle was in her fifties when she came to Dr. Nambudripad. She had cancer and knew she had to quit smoking. She smoked a pack a day and had been smoking since childhood. Though she had tried everything to quit, she had been unable to.

Muscle response testing revealed the usual sugar and B-complex allergies. Dr. Nambudripad cleared her of those allergies first and started her on extra vitamin-B complex in addition to Estelle's regular multivitamin.

The next step was to treat her allergy to cigarettes, which required two NAET sessions. In the first one, Estelle needed to be cleared of the allergy to tobacco itself, that is, to have her system reprogrammed through NAET so it would no longer regard tobacco as an allergen. In the second one, she needed to be cleared of an allergy to cigarette smoke. For the first, she held a vial with a tobacco sample. For the second, she needed to bring in the brand that she smoked, light up, and smell its smoke as it burned while Dr. Nambudripad gave her an NAET treatment. You have to clear an allergy to the smell, she explains, adding that it is the same with a perfume allergy. You can't just clear the allergy to the perfume; you also have to clear the smell of the perfume.

"After three treatments, she never touched a cigarette again," Dr. Nambudripad recalls. The addiction subsided naturally. Estelle no longer had any desire for a cigarette, despite the fact that she had been smoking most of her life. That was ten years ago, and Estelle has remained a nonsmoker. Fortunately, her cancer is in remission, and she is grateful for this second chance.

Bridget: Hidden Addiction

Bridget, a 26-year-old movie actress, came to Dr. Nambudripad for treatment of severe sinusitis. Through the question-and-response process of NAET muscle testing, it became clear that the sinusitus was a chronic problem caused by something she was smelling regularly. Bridget was unforthcoming as to what that might be. When the testing repeated this conclusion and Dr. Nambudripad told Bridget that she didn't want to press but treatment would not be successful unless she knew what to treat, Bridget finally admitted that what she had been "smelling" might be cocaine. She snorted it at least two or three times a week, often more, and had been doing so since she was 17. The sinusitis had developed soon after the onset of her cocaine use.

MRT revealed that she was allergic to cocaine. The sinusitis was an allergic reaction and disappeared after she was cleared of her cocaine allergy (along with the classic sugar and B-complex allergies).

As with cigarettes, Dr. Nambudripad notes that with drugs that are inhaled, it is necessary to clear the person for the smell of the drug as well as the substance of the drug. This requires that the person inhale the smell one more time, in the office, while undergoing NAET treatment to clear any allergy to the smell. As Dr. Nambudripad does not keep the actual drugs in her office, but only the energetic samples of each drug (meaning that the test vial does not contain biochemical traces but rather an energetic imprint of the substance), Bridget had to bring in a tiny amount of cocaine to sniff.

Due to the chronic nature of her addiction, it took five treatments to clear her of her allergy to cocaine. It has now been four years since her NAET treatment and Bridget is still off cocaine and free of sinusitis.

Gary: Marijuana Allergy and Pain

When Gary came to Dr. Nambudripad, he was in his thirties and had been suffering from spinal stenosis for the past six years. This is a progressive condition characterized by narrowing of the spinal canal, which compresses nerves and produces neck and back pain. Though he was still in the early stages of the illness, he had terrible neck and back pain, which was unusual as severe pain generally occurs in the later stages. To help reduce the pain, his doctor had given him Marinol, known as prescription marijuana because it is synthetic THC, which is the active compound in marijuana. "Medical marijuana," in the form of Marinol or the actual herb ingested or smoked, helps reduce nausea, improve appetite, and relieve pain and has proven beneficial in the case of cancer, AIDS, glaucoma, chronic pain, and multiple sclerosis, among other conditions.

The pain-relieving properties of THC did nothing for Gary's pain, however. It was the search for something to ease this severe discomfort that brought him to Dr. Nambudripad for treatment.

With his level of pain, Dr. Nambudripad expected to find quite a few allergies when she tested him, as allergies and their attendant inflammation contribute to any pain condition. But that was not the case. Upon questioning him, she learned about the Marinol and also the fact that Gary had been a regular marijuana smoker before the spinal stenosis began. After she cleared him for an allergy to marijuana, as well as the standard sugar and B-complex allergies, and started him on B-complex supplements, his neck and back pain subsided.

While Gary was likely allergic to marijuana before his doctor gave him Marinol, as evidenced by his level of pain, his case raises an important point, which is that many people are allergic to prescription (and even over-the-counter) drugs. "These people can be treated with NAET to remove the allergy to the drug and will then be able to use the drug without any reactions," states Dr. Nambudripad. "Sick patients may not have to go through unpleasant drug reactions and other aftereffects of the drugs."

While Gary was likely allergic to marijuana before his doctor gave him Marinol, as evidenced by his level of pain, his case raises an important point, which is that many people are allergic to prescription (and even over-the-counter) drugs.

In her patient intake questionnaire, Dr. Nambudripad has since added the question: "Do you use any drugs?" In her practice, she has found that hidden drug use, as in the cases of Gary and Bridget, with the associated allergies to those drugs, is often behind a range of otherwise unexplained symptoms, including pain.

In Gary's case, he also needed to be cleared for allergies to calcium and other minerals so he could properly absorb these nutrients. "Spinal stenosis is a condition of calcification," explains Dr. Nambudripad, adding that enabling the proper absorption of minerals would stop the progression of his condition.

Two years later Gary is still free of pain, and his spinal stenosis does not seem to be progressing. He has discovered that his pain returns if he eats something to which he is allergic. Having learned from Dr. Nambudripad how to check for allergies before eating, he is able for the most part to avoid this.

5 Energy Medicine I: Traditional Chinese Medicine

From the perspective of traditional Chinese medicine (TCM), any disorder, including addiction, results from a disturbance in energy flow in the body. That disturbance produces effects in the person's mind and spirit as well as on the physical level because body, mind, and spirit are inseparable, says Ira J. Golchehreh, L.Ac., O.M.D., whose practice is based in San Rafael, California.

All three operate on energy and are fed by the same source, so all three are impacted when the energy becomes imbalanced, he explains. By restoring proper energy flow in the body, TCM treatment thus helps restore balance in mind and spirit as well as body.

Many people in the West do not understand that traditional Chinese medicine, of which acupuncture is a component, is a complex system and requires as rigorous, if not more rigorous, training as Western medicine in order to be practiced correctly. The programs at the better traditional Chinese medical schools take eight years to complete. Dr. Golchehreh is a master of TCM, having trained with professors from the Shanghai Medical School, which is considered the Harvard Medical School of Chinese medicine. He has treated tens of thousands of patients in the 20 years that he has been practicing and can reverse many intractable conditions that other forms of medicine have been unable to treat.

While every individual is unique, certain meridians typically require treatment in cases of addiction, Dr. Golchehreh says. Before we turn to that, let's get a better understanding of TCM and the energy it addresses.

What Is Traditional Chinese Medicine?

Traditional Chinese medicine was developed over five thousand years ago in China and is still the predominant medical system used in that country today. It is also now widely practiced in the United States and other Western countries. The primary treatment modalities of TCM are acupuncture and Chinese herbal medicine. TCM is a form of energy, or vibrational, medicine, in that it is based on the flow of vital energy (*qi,* pronounced *chee*) in the body along energy channels known as meridians.

Another term for energy medicine is "molecular medicine," says Dr. Golchehreh. "When you look at the human being, you have to look at the molecular biology, the energy flow in the body, and the energy that is causing the vibrational weight between the cells and tissues."

Energy travels through the body along the meridians, which supply energy to organs, nerves, and other tissue. As explained in the previous chapter, there are 12 primary meridians relating to the organs or organ systems; each bears the name of the main organ it supplies, as in the Lung meridian, Heart meridian, Liver meridian, and Large Intestine meridian. In addition, there are two general meridians, the Governing Vessel and the Conception Vessel, as well as subsidiary energy channels. (See meridian charts on pages 86 and 87.)

Imbalances in energy flow can be excesses, deficiencies, or stagnation, and affect organs and systems throughout the body. TCM describes these imbalances and the attendant disharmony in the body in terms of natural world attributes such as heat, fire, cold, dampness, or dryness. These reflect the dominance of one or the other of the two essential qualities of qi: yin and yang. Yin is watery, dark, and calming, while yang is fiery, bright, and energizing. The names TCM uses to describe health conditions often have a poetic ring to them, as in Upflaming of Deficient Fire and Disorders of the Spirit Gate.

The flow of energy in the body can be thrown out of balance—become excessive, deficient, blocked, or stagnant—by influences on the physical, psychological, or spiritual levels. Biochemical, functional, or metabolic factors can be involved. A poor diet, organ malfunction, toxicity, and stress all affect energy flow in the body, as does substance abuse.

Genetics may be a factor as well. You can inherit a tendency for your qi to be deficient (or in excess), Dr. Golchehreh notes. "That genetic tendency could go back centuries." This inheritance may set you up for developing an addiction as one way to compensate for the energy imbalance. Similarly, he adds, a family history of diabetes can make a person susceptible to abuse of alcohol, as the body seeks to compensate for abnormal blood sugar levels with the sugar that alcoholic beverages provide. In either case, this self-medication throws the energy off even more.

The factors that affect qi can be internal or external. Just as the body, mind, and spirit are related within a human being, human beings are also elements in the environment, states Dr. Golchehreh. "You're definitely under the influence of what's going on outside, physically, chemically, and in every other way. Your body chemistry has a tendency to fluctuate accordingly. We are not individual parts. We are a part of the whole. That's why the pollution in the air, for example, could also cause some kind of problems internally, in the lung, the heart, and the liver."

A doctor of Chinese medicine diagnoses the status of energy flow in a patient via the pulses (at the wrist), appearance of the tongue, and other physical indications (such as the state of the skin, the person's mien or demeanor, and how he or she moves) that practitioners are trained to observe. The term "pulses" as it is used in TCM does not refer to the Western medicine pulse that is a measure of heart rate, but rather to distinct pulses corresponding to the organs and meridians. The energy qualities of the various pulses (essentially one for each meridian) are described in language such as wiry, thready, choppy, rapid, slow, floating, tight, and slippery. The quality signals to the practitioner the energy status of the organ and meridian.

As treatment, acupuncture and Chinese herbs are administered to address the specific energy imbalances of the patient: to raise deficient energy, reduce excess energy, or remove blockages producing energy stagnation.

In acupuncture, thin needles are shallowly inserted into the skin at strategic points (acupoints) along the meridian(s) requiring treatment and left in place for an average of a half-hour. This is a painless procedure, and patients often fall asleep while the needles are doing their work.

As with other natural medicine modalities, TCM treatment involves layers of healing. Underneath the energy imbalances that are producing the presenting symptoms may be other energy imbalances that can be addressed once the "top" layer is removed, explains Dr. Golchehreh. What is presenting on top is the acute aspect, and what is underlying is the chronic. "So there are different layers of a problem that affect a person psychologically, mentally, and physically," he concludes.

The complexity of influences involved in disorders such as addiction makes it imperative to consider the person as a whole—body, mind, and spirit—in treatment, as TCM does.

Acupuncture has application to a broad range of conditions, but has become particularly known in the United States for its efficacy in treating pain, addiction, and asthma, as well as reducing the side effects of chemotherapy.[215]

In the United States, there are thousands of acupuncturists and doctors of traditional Chinese medicine. These medical practices require extensive training. Ask practitioners for information about their training and avoid those who have only taken a quick course. One organization that can help you locate an acupuncturist in your area is the National Certification Commission for Acupuncture and Oriental Medicine (NCCAOM), 11 Canal Center Plaza, Suite 300, Alexandria, VA 22314; tel: 703-548-9004; website: www.nccaom.org. The National Acupuncture Detoxification Association (NADA) trains health professionals in using acupuncture to treat substance abuse. Contact NADA, P.O. Box 1927, Vancouver, WA 98668-1927; 888-765-NADA or 360-254-0186; website: www.acudetox.com.

The TCM Approach to Addiction

In the field of addictions, acupuncture is perhaps best known for its treatment to help people stop smoking, but it is also widely used to treat substance abuse of all kinds and has proven effective in reducing addictive cravings and withdrawal symptoms. Research has shown that acupuncture produces good results when used during detoxification and as initial treatment of heroin or cocaine addiction.[216]

In addition to programs that use acupuncture as an adjunct therapy in the treatment of addiction, there are over 175 acupuncture-based chemical dependency programs in existence in the United States alone. One of these, the Lincoln Hospital Clinic in the South Bronx, New York, has been using acupuncture combined with traditional counseling to treat substance abuse since 1974. The clinic sees 250 people a day, among whom are the more than 1,000 people who are referred to the clinic every year by welfare and criminal justice agencies. The clinic's success rate, based on clean urine tests, is 60 percent of all users treated since the inception of the acupuncture program. Among the 8,000 crack patients, the urine tests of over 50 percent have come up clean for periods longer than two months.[217]

Auricular acupuncture (treatment via acupuncture points on the ears) has been the focus of a number of studies, typically for nicotine or cocaine addiction. Some researchers concluded that acupuncture is beneficial, while others concluded that it is not. The problem with these studies is that auricular acupuncture, which is used to reduce cravings, is only one aspect of the treatment of addiction when TCM is used correctly. To employ only the tool that reduces cravings is indicative of conventional medical thinking, which seeks a quick solution that doesn't address the deeper imbalances in a given condition or require the patient to do anything.

Yes, some people will be able to overcome their addiction only with assistance to reduce their cravings during the most difficult period just after quitting their substance of choice. These people obviously do not need to make major lifestyle changes or have acupuncture that treats deeper energy imbalances in order to kick their habit. This explains the positive research results.

The negative research results of studies that look only at auricular acupuncture, however, should not be interpreted as evidence that acupuncture does not work as a treatment for addictions. Studying only auricular treatment is like testing Band-Aids on serious wounds and concluding that first-aid intervention is of no use for injuries. Addiction is a complicated condition and for most people effective treatment must go further than reducing cravings.

"Auricular acupuncture is not the solution to the problem," says Dr. Golchehreh. "If the person has serious problems on the Lung, Heart, or Liver meridians, you have to identify and solve the problems. We use auricular acupuncture to complement the constitutional points (the points on the body along the primary meridians)."

Further, TCM treatment varies according to the individual. Along with constitutional factors, the person's age, the number of years of substance abuse, and the level of consumption all modify treatment. TCM places individuals who overuse substances in two distinct groups: those with substance abuse and those with substance dependency. Aside from individual factors, the difference in treatment is that with dependency treatment must alleviate withdrawal symptoms.

Dr. Golchehreh places abuse and dependency along a continuum from mild to severe. On the mild end, people can quit with only a little help and not go through intense withdrawal or need deep treatment to address damage wreaked by substance abuse. Those in the moderate category will have withdrawal symptoms when they quit, depending on their substance of choice, and are likely to need a moderate amount of treatment to restore the proper flow of energy along certain meridians and to detoxify their blood and organs. Those in the severe category are those whose substance abuse has been extreme or chronic. Their withdrawal symptoms are correspondingly severe, with attendant conditions such as instability, anger, depression, anxiety, restlessness, insomnia, and inability to concentrate.

While TCM can reduce withdrawal symptoms, stop cravings, and restore the proper flow of energy in the body, there are behavioral and lifestyle components to substance abuse and dependency that must be addressed for treatment to be successful. "Part of the problem with most people who are abusers or dependents is that it is not only that the body has the craving, but that there are also a whole set of behaviors that go with use of the substance," explains Dr. Golchehreh. "The person has to make behavioral changes."

Dr. Golchehreh points to two main reasons for a person's failure to quit. The first is that the practitioner doesn't know how to treat the substance abuse or addiction and fails to address the root problems. The second is that the patient does not change the behaviors associated with his substance abuse and so is unable to move out of the habit.

TCM can "kill the cravings for smoking in probably three or four visits," for instance, says Dr. Golchehreh, but then it is up to individuals to change their behavior or habits to support a nonsmoking way of life. In some cases, when the person is highly motivated to quit, as with the life-and-death situation facing William in the case to follow, one acupuncture treatment is all that's needed for the person to quit, but three to four is more typical for all substances. Then, more treatment may be advisable to undo the damage caused by the substance abuse.

> *"Part of the problem with most people who are abusers or dependents is that it is not only that the body has the craving, but that there are also a whole set of behaviors that go with use of the substance," explains Dr. Golchehreh. "The person has to make behavioral changes."*

Just as there is a continuum of degrees of substance abuse, there is a continuum of degrees of motivation to quit. In Dr. Golchehreh's practice, he notes three distinct groups. "Many people are ashamed and embarrassed and don't even want to talk about their addiction. Others come straight to me for treatment because they have done everything, and failed. The third group consists of those who come for treatment of other symptoms. They face that problem, and then they want to deal with their addiction." The third group makes up about 80 percent of those Dr. Golchehreh treats for substance abuse. They may come for treatment of a skin condition or neck pain or headaches, and in the course of treatment they become motivated to deal with their substance problem.

The Components of Treatment

The major components in TCM treatment of substance abuse or dependency are: the physical examination, educating the patient, controlling the craving and clearing the toxicity, dietary recommendations, and undoing the damage. At the same time, it is necessary for individuals to deal with the behavioral, psychological, and lifestyle aspects of their substance abuse.

The Physical Examination: What the Body Tells

The first step is a physical exam using the diagnostic measures described earlier. The physical parameters, however, give information on the state of the individual at all levels—physically, mentally, and spiritually. "I don't need to ask someone, 'How's your spiritual life?' The body tells me," explains Dr. Golchehreh. "For example, if I take the pulse and it is rapid and wiry, I know that this person has emotional problems. It's all written there for you when you know how to read it."

Indicators of substance abuse can be found in many physical attributes, including general appearance (lack of grooming, edgy motion), neurological disturbance (such as the lack of coordination caused by drug abuse), the state of the skin (profuse sweating, broken blood vessels on the face, flushed face), the state of the tongue (for example, the tongue is yellowish with a thick coating in those who abuse alcohol, while it is red with a thin coating in cases of drug abuse), the state of the pupils (enlarged), abdomen distension (from liver enlargement), and the quality of the pulses. For example, the pulse is superficial and rapid in those who abuse drugs, while with alcohol the quality of the pulse depends on the kind of alcohol consumed. With beer, it is more solid and rapid; with wine, more sedate and calm; and hard liquor tends to produce a mixture of both qualities.

The diagnostic signs range from mild to severe depending on how much the individual uses of a given substance, says Dr. Golchehreh. This information provides him with pieces of the puzzle, which when assembled points the way to the proper treatment. "Every case must be approached individually, taking into consideration the individual constitution."

Educating the Patient

The second step in TCM treatment of addiction is to educate the patient on the physical effects of the substance abuse in which they are engaged to underline the importance of quitting and provide facts to support their decision. In the case of smoking, for example, Dr. Golchehreh explains to them exactly what happens when they inhale the cigarette smoke, how the nicotine goes directly into the bloodstream and from there into the liver, along with all of the other toxic and carcinogenic compounds from the tobacco and cigarette filter.

He lists the diseases and health conditions it can cause, which include cancer, heart disease, stroke, and chronic obstructive pulmonary disease (COPD). Despite media enumeration of all the negatives of smoking and drug abuse, Dr. Golchehreh has found that most people have not truly taken in this information. "You would be shocked by how many people really don't know," says Dr. Golchehreh.

Controlling the Craving and Clearing the Toxicity

The next step is to control the craving and clear the toxicity that has resulted from the substance abuse. Dr. Golchehreh accomplishes this through acupuncture treatment involving ear points and constitutional points on the body, as well as herbal and homeopathic medicine. In the case of smoking, for example, the focus is on clearing the Lung, Heart, and Liver meridians, which helps clear the associated organs; with alcohol, the focus is on the Liver meridian.

Clearing the toxicity has a dual purpose. It lifts the load on the body and helps reduce craving. Again, in the case of smoking, nicotine mainly affects the lungs, heart, and liver. By clearing the main organs and meridians of nicotine, cravings are reduced, Dr. Golchehreh explains, adding that Chinese medicine has had excellent results with this approach.

In addition to constitutional (on the body) points, he uses the three important points on the ears that correspond with the three

TCM Treatment of Substance Abuse/Dependency

While TCM treatment is individualized, the following are often part of the protocol in cases of substance abuse.

Smokers

Acupuncture meridians/points: Lung, Heart, Gateway to Heaven points, ear points

Treatment: Clear the lungs, nourish the heart, and calm the spirit; herbs to tonify the yin, transform hot phlegm, cool the body, and ease the cough

Herbs: radix peucedani, fructus trichosanthis, bulbus fritillariae, thallus algae, concha cyclinae sinensis, herba sargasii, semen sterculiae scaphigarae

Other remedies: homeopathic anti-smoking drops

Drug Abusers/Dependents

Acupuncture meridians/points: Heart, Liver, Lung, Spleen, ear points

Treatment: Quell the fire, cool the blood, calm the spirit, and nourish the heart; herbs to extinguish wind, stop tremors, and open the orifices

Herbs: os draconis, concha ostreae, margarita, succinum, haematitum, semen zizphi spinosae

Other remedies: homeopathic substance abuse drops

Alcohol Abusers/Dependents

Acupuncture meridians/points: Heart, Liver, Spleen, ear points

Treatment: Clean and detoxify the liver, cool the blood, clear the heat and poisons, tonify the blood, and tonify the yin; herbs to settle and calm the spirit, nourish the heart, and open the orifices

Herbs: cornu rhinoceri, radix rehmanniae, radix scrophulariae, cortex moutan radicis

Other remedies: homeopathic substance abuse drops

organs. "The ear is not on the constitutional system. It has to do with the vagus nerve, which is the tenth cranial nerve. The vagus nerve supplies and nourishes all the organs in the body. The only place where it comes to the surface of the body is at the ear." The concept of auricular (ear) acupuncture is that those points are related to the organs, and treating those points corrects the function of the corresponding organ.

"For example, if you use the liver point, it is going to clear the function of the liver, or if you use the lung point, it is going to help the lung. But that does not cover it," Dr. Golchehreh emphasizes. As discussed earlier, the ear points and constitutional points must be used in combination.

He advises against using nicotine patches to try to quit smoking because they put more nicotine into the bloodstream, affect kidney function, and can cause a range of physical problems, including high blood pressure, hyperthyroidism (an overactive thyroid gland), ulcers, and fertility problems. "Chinese medicine is a purer way to quit smoking," he concludes.

Herbal medicine is an important part of TCM treatment. The herbs prescribed again depend on the individual and the type of substance abuse. Dr. Golchehreh also uses homeopathic remedies to help clear toxicity and control craving, specifically anti-smoking drops or substance abuse drops, which are combination formulas that can be taken orally whenever craving arises. Like the acupuncture treatment, the remedies help to purify the organs implicated in the different types of abuse. Among the ingredients in the substance abuse drops are homeopathic *Valeriana, Avena sativa, Nux vomica, Tabacum, Coffea,* Endorphins, and *Absinthium*; in the anti-smoking drops are Adrenal, Kidney, Lung, and Endorphin preparations, along with *Nux vomica, Tabacum,* and *Nicotinum,* among others.

Dietary Recommendations

Certain dietary practices support the quitting process. "The change of a diet is very, very important for a couple of days. If they can handle 48 hours, this program usually works very well," Dr. Golchehreh says. He advises his patients to eat light meals like soup versus heavy foods, stay away from greasy or spicy foods, drink lots of pure water to help flush out the system, and avoid alcohol (even if it is not the substance one is trying to quit). These practices reduce the load on the body. "The greasy and spicy foods also create a craving for smoking," he notes, as does alcohol consumption.

Eating vegetables that aid in detoxification, especially ones that clean the liver, such as cauliflower, is helpful. Mint made into tea and mixed with food is another good liver cleanser, while cabbage and green peppers help break down viscous (thick) blood, notes Dr. Golchehreh.

If one is trying to overcome an alcohol problem, it is important to replace the sugar that it provides to the body. Maintaining a good blood sugar level helps to prevent cravings. Carbohydrates, fruit, and grape, orange, and other fruit juices are good dietary choices for this.

As in all TCM treatment, diet is tailored to individuals, depending on their constitution. Even though they may share the same addiction, the treatment details may be different. For example, someone who is heavy and has an enlarged liver needs a different diet from someone who is slim and has a normal liver, though both suffer from alcoholism, notes Dr. Golchehreh. "While it is important to adjust the diet to the individual constitution, it is also important to keep in mind that the person is going through a big change in habits and sacrificing a big desire, so it is necessary to be gentle and not push them too hard." To that end, he usually recommends just adding a couple of the previously mentioned foods to the diet.

Undoing the Damage

Substance abuse of any duration damages the body in some way. Acupuncture and herbal medicine can help reverse these effects. The degree and longevity of the abuse, as well as the individual's constitution, determine how much treatment will be needed to undo the damage, or reduce the effects if the damage to organs is too extensive to undo.

In alcohol and drug abuse, the liver is typically the organ most affected, while with smoking, as noted earlier, it is the lungs, heart, and liver. But the effects are wide-reaching. Substance abuse can create energy imbalances on any or all of the meridians. A number of drugs, for example, produce abnormalities in the meridians that cause tremors or shivering. Drugs and other substances also create energy blockages in what are known in TCM as the body's orifices, which include the brain, the chest, and the abdominal and other body cavities. For instance, in alcohol abuse, the orifice typically implicated is the abdominal cavity because the liver is affected and in turn produces extensive blockage in the whole area.

Herbs and acupuncture are used to clear the energy blockages in organs and orifices. The particular Chinese herbal medicines used depend upon the nature of the damage, as determined by the diagnostic tools discussed earlier in the chapter.

In more severe alcohol dependency, Dr. Golchehreh works "to clear the blood in general to help the organ that is damaged" and prescribes purging herbs to clean the system. Rhizoma rhei is one that works especially well on the liver, large intestines, and stomach. Aloe vera cleans the liver, spleen, stomach, and large intestines. "Because the liver is so toxic, and also because it's so full of the heat and the fire, we try to clear the heat and purge the fire," he says. "For this, *Gypsum fibrosum* and *Plumula nelumbinis* are excellent."

> **In more severe alcohol dependency, Dr. Golchehreh works "to clear the blood in general to help the organ that is damaged" and prescribes purging herbs to clean the system. Rhizoma rhei is one that works especially well on the liver, large intestines, and stomach. Aloe vera cleans the liver, spleen, stomach, and large intestines.**

Not everyone completes this portion of treatment. Some people are satisfied once they have quit their substance of choice. Others want to pursue treatment to undo the damage done by their former habit. For example, one longtime smoker was recently able to stop smoking after only one treatment, but she is continuing treatment with Dr. Golchehreh to "open" her lungs and clear her Heart meridian. "Clear" as it is used in TCM means to restore the proper energy flow on a given meridian. Restoring the energy flow enhances the function of the associated organ. In the case of this former smoker's lungs, more work was needed to open her lungs, that is, to return them to full function.

The Behavioral, Psychological, and Lifestyle Component

As discussed earlier, TCM treatment can go far in ending addiction, but without the patient addressing the behavioral, psychological, and lifestyle issues that support substance abuse, treatment is unlikely to be successful on a lasting basis. Herbal medicine can provide support for dealing with the psychological and emotional aspects, however. For example, when depression is an issue, Dr. Golchehreh has found that hypericin (the active ingredient in St. John's wort) can provide effective relief, as can kava-kava for anxiety.

His approach has successfully ended substance abuse of all kinds. When it has failed, it is generally because the person was unable to make the behavioral, psychological, or lifestyle changes necessary to end the habit. "I have no control over what they do when they leave the office. I tell them, 'That part is up to you. If you want to get the results, you need to make the changes. If you don't want it, that's a different story.'"

To get the support they need for making those changes and for processing what they are going through as they try to quit drugs or alcohol in particular, Dr. Golchehreh recommends a support group and/or a psychotherapist or psychologist. This is especially important for young people, he notes.

The following cases demonstrate the effectiveness of traditional Chinese medicine in helping people overcome substance abuse.

William: 50 Years of Smoking

William was 74 years old and had been smoking two to three packs a day for 50 years when he came to Dr. Golchehreh for help in quitting. He had emphysema, which had progressed to the point that he was on oxygen and had to have a tank with him at all times. He would stop the oxygen for cigarette breaks. His family was appalled. He was ready to quit, knowing that his smoking was killing him, but had tried repeatedly and been unable to do so on his own.

His lungs were extremely weak. "Emphysema causes the balloon-type lung, which means that the lung is wide open and loses its elasticity," says Dr. Golchehreh. "It's not opening and closing correctly. The air is trapped in the lung, so you have to push the air out of the lungs to improve the elasticity." He addressed this with acupuncture and recommended Herba mentha to relieve the pressure in the lungs and help clear the Liver meridian.

Otherwise, Dr. Golchehreh followed the classic protocol for

quitting smoking. He treated the constitutional and ear points, gave William the typical herbs (see sidebar) along with the usual dietary recommendations for the withdrawal period, and instructed him to take three drops of the homeopathic anti-smoking drops whenever he felt the craving for a cigarette. He told William that he could come back for further acupuncture treatment if he was having a hard time.

"This patient was so eager to quit smoking that he did everything I told him to do," recalls Dr. Golchehreh. "In his case, all it took was that one acupuncture treatment, followed by observing the protocol I had given him." Of course, William still had emphysema, but the state of his lungs was improved, and he was no longer smoking.

Susan: Out-of-Control Drinking

Susan, 56, had a high-profile, high-responsibility job. She was very efficient and good at what she did, but she felt great stress from the demands of work and the burden of responsibility she carried. She started drinking at the end of the day to calm her down. As time went on, the amount she drank every night increased steadily, despite her best efforts to cut back. She started having anxiety attacks and only found relief when she drank. When her performance at work began to suffer, she realized that the problem was beyond her and she needed to get some help. She checked into first one rehabilitation center and then another, but each time she began drinking again shortly after leaving the center.

"These programs failed because they did not get to the root of the problem," observes Dr. Golchehreh, to whom Susan came in desperation. By the time she sought his help, she had been drinking heavily for several years. After the initial consultation, he determined that Susan's treatment needed to happen in stages.

The first step was to calm her nervous system, which would alleviate her anxiety attacks and reduce her level of fear. Dr. Golchehreh devoted the first acupuncture treatment to accomplishing this through a combination of ear points and constitutional points on the body. The ear points would also help stop her craving for alcohol. In addition, he sent Susan home with a form of acupuncture needles known as staples installed in her ears. Despite their name, these don't involve piercing the ear. Like other acupuncture needles, they are painless. They don't show and can be left in place between treatments, where they continue their rebalancing work and help to kill cravings.

The second step was to detoxify Susan's liver through acupuncture points and herbal medicine, notably an herbal liver cleanse, which contains dandelion, beetroot, milk thistle, cascara, parsley, licorice root, bearberry, nettle roots, and picorrhiza. Susan later reported that after this second session, she stopped drinking and lost her craving for alcohol as well. In the third session, Dr. Golchehreh focused on constitutional points to restore balance to Susan's body, mind, and spirit and on continuing to clear her liver.

Early in treatment, he had started her on the herbal drops specifically designed for substance abuse and recommended that she drink lots of grape and other fruit juices to keep her blood sugar levels up and thus reduce her craving for alcohol. As Susan normally ate a diet high in animal protein and her pulses revealed that her blood was viscous, Dr. Golchehreh recommended that she eat foods that help break down the viscosity of the blood, such as green peppers and cabbage.

"People who are vegetarian don't usually have a problem with alcohol," he notes. Their blood is less viscous, so flows more normally, than that of people who eat a heavier diet. With a diet that emphasizes animal proteins, the viscosity of the blood changes, becomes heavier. These people may unconsciously turn to alcohol in an attempt to reduce the viscosity, to get their blood flowing better, says Dr. Golchehreh.

In Susan's case, she desperately wanted to get rid of her drinking problem, but the addiction was in her blood—literally. "We had to change the quality of the viscosity of the blood in order to get results," explains Dr. Golchehreh. "Rehab works for some people, but it doesn't work for others. One reason is that they don't look at the quality of the blood."

He reiterates that every individual is different and requires slightly different treatment. In Susan's case, the main components of treatment were to calm her nervous system, change the quality of the viscosity of her blood, and cleanse her liver, in addition to treating her craving and keeping her blood sugar levels up during her withdrawal from alcohol.

Dr. Golchehreh gave Susan acupuncture treatments weekly for a total of nine sessions. Five months later, she is still off alcohol and no longer suffers from anxiety attacks. Though her job is as stressful as ever, she is better able to cope with it.

6 Energy Medicine II:
Flower Essence Therapy

Like traditional Chinese medicine, flower essence therapy works on an energetic level to restore the equilibrium of the body, mind, and spirit. The particular specialty of flower essences is the realm of emotions and attitudes, which exert a powerful influence on health and ill health. As Edward Bach, an English physician and homeopath and the father of flower essence therapy, stated it, "Behind all disease lie our fears, our anxieties, our greed, our likes and dislikes."[219] By addressing underlying psychospiritual issues and promoting energetic shifts in the mind and emotions, flower essences promote a return to health on all levels.

Put simply, flower essences are "catalysts to mind-body wellness," explains Patricia Kaminski, codirector of the Flower Essence Society in Nevada City, California, and a renowned innovator in the field of flower essence therapy for over 20 years (see "What Is Flower Essence Therapy?"). Or you could say they act as a bridge between the realms of the physical and the spiritual, the body and the soul.[220]

Every disorder, including addiction, contains a lesson for the person afflicted. From the viewpoint of flower essence therapy, this lesson regards a psychospiritual or soul issue that is not being dealt with or a psychospiritual need that is not being met, says Kaminski. These neglected areas of the individual create energy imbalances that over time can manifest in illness. By helping to bring psychospiritual issues

In Their Own Words

"I would draw addiction as a tree, with the branches being alcoholism, codependency, over-eating, etc. Each manifestation needs separate attention, but at root they are the same process of spiritual separation."
—a person in recovery[221]

and unmet needs to light, flower essences facilitate the resolution of these issues, rebalancing of the attendant energy disturbances, and restoration of health.

A purely biochemical model fails to address the emotional, psychological, and spiritual components of addiction. If brain chemistry is skewed, what caused that to happen? According to the flower essence model, the biochemical imbalances found in addiction are caused by the distress of the spirit, or soul, says Kaminski. Thus, a purely biochemical approach will not cure addiction because it does not deal with the source—the soul's crisis.

The embracing of the biochemical model in medicine reflects our cultural bias for physical development over psychospiritual development, she observes. For example, exercising the body to develop its strength or undergoing physical therapy to redevelop strength after a stroke or an injury are standard and widespread practices. But a similar emphasis on psychospiritual development in "mental disorders" is lacking. Instead, medical intervention seeks to remove the symptoms as quickly as possible. "We intervene earlier and earlier when someone is in emotional pain and distress," states Kaminski. "We use biochemical therapies to 'fix' the problem at its current level of symptom manifestation, rather than encouraging further psychological development."

This is where flower essences can be a valuable tool. "The approach of flower essence therapy is to recognize the dignity of the human soul and to recognize the capacity of the human soul to change and become stronger," she elaborates. "The soul isn't connected to the aging of the body, so even if you're 70 years old, you can still be developing from the point of view of the soul. What we want to look at when somebody is facing a crisis, when they present with anxiety, with depression, with an addiction, is what is it that the soul is really facing. . . . There's enormous capacity in the human spirit and the human soul to acquire skills for transforming what is a problem into a gift, if the therapy goes deep enough."

What Is Flower Essence Therapy?

The use of flower essences is often dismissed in the United States, even by some alternative medicine practitioners, as a "lightweight" therapy that may be pleasing but has little therapeutic value. In actuality, flower essence therapy has the capability to stimulate profound change on a deep level. One reason for the misconception may be the general lack of understanding in this country about energy medicine, which is widely accepted in Europe. As the promising results of scientific investigation into flower essence therapy and other forms of energy medicine are mounting and an increasing number of alternative medicine physicians and other healthcare professionals are routinely employing these modalities, the misconceptions are gradually being dispelled. More people are discovering the truth about flower essence therapy, which is that it has the capability to stimulate profound change on a deep level, Kaminski states.

To clarify another common misunderstanding, essential oils (aromatherapy) and flower essences are two very different kinds of medicine. While essential oils contain the biochemical components of the plants from which they are extracted, flower essences are closer to homeopathic remedies in nature, in that they are energetic imprints of their source. Another way of saying this is that a flower essence contains the life force of the flower.

A flower essence is made by sun-infusing the blossoms of a particular plant, bush, or tree in water. (This is a simplistic summary of the process, which involves timing the picking of the flowers according to life-cycle, environmental, and other factors.) The liquid is then diluted and potentized in a method similar to the preparation of homeopathic remedies and preserved with brandy (or a nonalcoholic substance, if need be). The result is a highly diluted, potentized substance that embodies the energetic patterns of the flower from which it is made. This means that the therapeutic effects of flower essences are vibrational or energetic.[222]

Despite Einstein and solid science demonstrating that matter is energy, the fact that you can contain energy in a liquid and influence human energy fields to help resolve ailments is not widely known. Yet, that is precisely what flower essence liquids do. When you take flower essences, the energy they contain affects your energy field, which in turn has an impact on your physical, mental, emotional, and spiritual condition, as these aspects are all energy based.

In the 1930s, Dr. Bach, an English physician and homeopath, developed 38 different flower essences to address 38 different emotional-soul or psychological types. As an example of the "profile" associated with a remedy, the flower essence Willow is indicated for someone who, when out of balance, feels resentful, bitter, and envious of others and adopts a "poor me" victim stance. Dr. Bach's remedies are still available today as the Bach Flower Remedies seen in health food stores everywhere.

The Flower Essence Society (FES) in Nevada City, California, headed by Kaminski and her husband, Richard Katz, has expanded on the work of Dr. Bach and significantly furthered the field of flower essences. Founded in 1979 by Katz, FES is a pioneer in flower essence research, compiling and analyzing case study data from tens of thousands of practitioners worldwide and conducting longitudinal studies as well as botanical field studies.

FES also funds double-blind placebo trials with specific flower essences. In two such studies, clinical and research psychologist Jeffrey Cram, Ph.D., director of the Sierra Health Institute in Nevada City, looked at the efficacy of specific flower essence formulas in alleviating stress. Physiological measures showed significantly reduced reactivity in subjects who received the flower essences versus those given a placebo.[223] Currently under way is a major study on the application of flower essences in depression.[224]

In addition to the society's involvement in research, Kaminski and Katz expanded on Bach's remedies, developing a line of more than 100 flower essences derived from North American plants. They developed the line (the FES brand) to expand the emotional repertoire of flower essences; to provide North Americans with essences derived from indigenous plants, which might better resonate with their healing issues; and to address the more complicated emotional and psychological makeup of people today.

 There are many flower essence practitioners. **The Flower Essence Society operates a Practitioner Referral Network, with a listing of about 3,000 flower essence therapists in the U.S. and Canada alone; contact Flower Essence Society, P.O. Box 459, Nevada City, CA 95959; tel: 530-265-9163 or 800-736-9222; website: www.flower society.org.**

The Soul Message in Addiction

"Addiction is a human longing," says Kaminski. "We all experience pain in some way. We all experience incompleteness in some way. We all seek some substance or some experience that will give us relief from our pain, some way that we can become whole again. The point is, is the addiction ruling us? How dysfunctional are we around the addiction?"

A medical model that acknowledges that we all have some capacity for addiction, that the soul longs for wholeness and connection, focuses on identifying what the soul of an individual is missing and what can be done to fill that hole from within. From the point of view of a flower essence therapist, physical aspects of addiction, such as biochemical imbalances, are caused by the soul's distress, our psychospiritual needs. "The brain is a receptor and a reflector for what is happening with our souls," states Kaminski.

Flower essence therapy facilitates the process of answering the soul's needs from within. The flower essences used depend upon the nature of the soul's longing, says Kaminski. "With addiction, you have every known human suffering. Every addiction tells a story about the soul, and we can't just say, 'Here, take this for addiction.'"

The first therapeutic step then is to identify the nature of the soul's pain. For this information, Kaminski asks clients about their dreams, has them draw, and talks on a deep level with them. Dreams and drawing reflect the content of the subconscious and often reveal what a person may not be aware or cannot put into words. What

117

Kaminski learns indicates which flower essences will be useful in each individual case. While everyone is unique, the following sections delineate the soul messages that Kaminski has found are often associated with specific types of addiction, as well as the flower essences that have proven useful in the corresponding soul healing.

Alcohol

The soul pain in alcoholism is most often "a well of loneliness . . . a profound loneliness," observes Kaminski. The soul longing is for love and connection. Alcohol takes the place of that, which explains the assertion from many alcoholics that the bottle is their best friend. Kaminski points to this soul longing as the reason why Twelve-Step programs are so effective for alcoholics. "They're not as effective for a number of other addictions, but they're particularly effective in alcoholism. They provide a social context for people, give them a group."

The flower essences needed are those that "nourish the capacity of the soul to feel social warmth, not to have to feel it from the fire of alcohol, but to feel the fire of the heart." Remedies such as Mallow, Goldenrod, and Holly are useful for this and help the person to feel loved and to express love.

Black-Eyed Susan is also frequently indicated to promote self-healing and to help work through all the levels of denial. Kaminski notes that denial is deep, even when people acknowledge that they have a problem and seek help to overcome it. "You need remedies, first of all, to start breaking the addiction, to give them the courage to do that."

Tobacco

With cigarettes, the soul pain is avoidance of painful or uncomfortable emotions, notes Kaminski. Smoking provides an emotional mask, a "smokescreen" to hide buried issues with which the heart hasn't dealt. (Heart in this sense is the emotional heart rather than the organ or the meridian, discussed in the previous chapter.) "This may be the case with alcohol, too, but there's something about cigarette addiction that is more insidious. Every alcoholic I've ever met knows they're in trouble. But while people who smoke cigarettes know that it isn't good for their health, they are shocked to find out how emotionally messed up they are when they try to quit smoking. It's a major revelation for them."

This may be why it is one of the hardest addictions to overcome. Lighting up a cigarette can help a person avoid feeling. "In the classic cliché, the couple makes love and the man lights up a cigarette afterwards. That way, he doesn't have to deal too much with anything tender." Cigarette ads reflect this truth, notes Kaminski, as epitomized by the Marlboro man with his tough, leathery face, alone and self-sufficient in a rugged landscape that hearkens back to the Old West. Cigarettes and soldiers are also inextricably linked, with the U.S. military until recently providing free or cheap cigarettes to enlisted personnel.

Many people who suffer from anxiety are smokers. While nicotine actually speeds the body up, it paradoxically has a calming effect on the smoker. When someone begins to feel anxious over an argument, criticism from the boss, or other daily life event that raises anxiety, lighting up a cigarette becomes a way to cope with it. "When you stop smoking, you then have to deal with emotions, and this is what makes it so hard to quit," says Kaminski.

With smoking and other forms of tobacco addiction, the flower essence indicated to start with is typically Nicotiana, one of the purest existing strains of the actual tobacco plant. This is an important remedy for the heart, in the emotional sense. The pattern of imbalance it addresses is "numbing of the emotions" and "inability to cope with deep feelings."[225] Another commonly used essence, depending on the person, is Yerba Santa, which means in Spanish "holy herb." This essence is indicated for lung conditions, both physical and emotional. Constricted feelings in the chest are an example of the latter. The patterns of imbalance it addresses are these constricted feelings and "deeply repressed emotions."[226]

Borage, which promotes "ebullient heart forces," can also be important, states Kaminski, "to release all the congestion in the heart and lung area. That's the main area where repressed emotions are stored." In addition, flower essence therapists often use Chaparral in the initial stages to pull the "psychic and physical toxicity" from the body.[227]

It should be noted that from an energy perspective the physical is inseparable from the psychospiritual. Held emotions, for example, produce tightness in the body and interfere with the flow of energy in the traditional Chinese medicine sense, so the organs in the area where repressed emotions are stored will be affected.

People who are trying to stop smoking need assistance, especially during the first week, in dealing with the emotions that come up, as they are no longer held down by the smoking. "Some people have an overwhelming amount of anxiety," says Kaminski. For them, Five-Flower Formula (also known as Rescue Remedy) or other flower essences that promote calm are indicated. For other people, anger is the primary emotion that surfaces. These are people who, instead of expressing their anger, would have a cigarette. There are many flower essences to help with anger. While the emotional content and therefore the flower essence indicated vary among individuals in the first stages of quitting, the common denominator, states Kaminski, "is that with every single person who detoxes from cigarettes, there is a lot of emotional toxicity."

Cocaine and Other Stimulants

In cases of addiction to stimulants such as cocaine, "the soul is longing for the sense of the life force," to feel filled with the energy of life, Kaminski explains. Ironically, the means by which stimulant addicts attempt to fulfill that longing will, over time, rob them of energy, as these drugs burn out the adrenal and other systems in the body designed to give us energy.

One of the primary flower essences indicated for addiction to stimulants is Morning Glory, which helps restore the balanced rhythm of day and night. "People who are addicted to stimulants are usually night owls who have a hard time getting up in the morning and need stimulants to keep their energy up during the day. Morning Glory helps to start reversing the flow, so they can feel more and more real life energy." Other flower essences are used as indicated in individual cases to facilitate self-healing and get people back "to feeling life on its own terms rather than pushing the physical reality," explains Kaminski.

Heroin

With heroin addiction, the presenting symptom is a desire to escape from life, almost an indifference to life, says Kaminski. The soul is "longing for light, longing for Heaven on Earth." The ecstasy of a heroin high temporarily assuages that longing and makes the user never want to come back to normal reality. "That's why it's such a powerful addiction," she says.

To help the individual overcome heroin addiction, one of the main flower essences used is California Poppy, which is from the same family as the Oriental poppy, the source of opium, which in turn contains the alkaloids heroin and morphine. California Poppy helps people begin "to experience light as a force in their heart, but a light that makes them want to be here on Earth, not out of body." The imbalance that it addresses is "seeking outside oneself for false forms of light or higher consciousness, especially through escapism or addiction."[228]

Marijuana and Hallucinogenic Drugs

In abuse of marijuana and hallucinogenic drugs such as LSD, peyote, psilocybin mushrooms, and ayahuasca, the soul is longing for transcendent spiritual experiences and expansion of consciousness. "However, the soul ultimately becomes weakened because the spiritual forces are not developed incrementally from within the innate spiritual strength of the soul," states Kaminski. "While initial insights and experiences can be gained, ultimately such drugs are a crutch and work against the free spiritual creativity and independence of the soul."

Flower essences to help ground "the structures of light" within the individual and to help that person "see through false spiritual or illusory experiences" are California Poppy, Angelica, Lotus, Star Tulip, Alpine Aster, Cosmos, Shasta Daisy, St. John's Wort, Mountain Pennyroyal, and Angel's Trumpet.

Food

With food addiction, people are eating to replace or to numb out emotions, states Kaminski. She cites four predominant emotional syndromes in cases of food addiction: shielding and protecting; numbing and stuffing; social paralysis; and stress and strain.

Shielding and Protecting: With the soul in a state of heightened vulnerability and sensitivity, the person uses eating as a way to cope with hypersensitivity and weight as a kind of armor and protection. Weight is often distributed in emotionally sensitive areas of the body, such as the abdomen, hips, and torso in general (protecting the heart, solar plexus, and pelvis). Childhood trauma such as sexual or physical abuse may be a factor in the disposition toward shielding and protecting. "Many women practice some degree of shielding around the more emotionally vulnerable time before their menstrual cycles, with temporary gains in weight or water retention," notes Kaminski. "The key to healing the shielding response is to create an inner sense of security and psychic containment," she states. "Such individuals also need to come into greater levels of trust regarding their bodies and the physical and emotional environment surrounding them."

In this syndrome of food addiction, indicated flower essences, depending on the individual, are Yarrow, Pink Yarrow, Golden Yarrow, and Yarrow Environmental Formula (YES, and FES formulation), Pink Monkeyflower, Sticky Monkeyflower, Hibiscus, Chamomile, Dill, Angelica, and St. John's Wort.

Numbing and Stuffing: This type of emotional syndrome turns to eating as a means of numbing or temporarily obliterating conscious awareness. Addiction to other numbing drugs such as alcohol may also be in evidence. The soul longing is to be free of painful emotions, which are buried or repressed. Bulimia is an extreme manifestation of this syndrome. "The key to successful recovery from stuffing and numbing behavior is to retrieve emotional memory and awareness," states Kaminski. "Also highly important is that the individual integrate the shadow or hidden part of the self that resists coming to the light of awareness."

The flower essences that can help with this syndrome are Black-Eyed Susan, Agrimony, Milkweed, Golden Ear Drops, Fuchsia, Chocolate Lily, and Star of Bethlehem.

Social Paralysis: This syndrome is formed by internalized social, cultural, religious, or familial attitudes toward food, eating, and weight. Those in this category are unable to perceive themselves as they are, and weight can range from anorexic to obese. The soul longing is to return to a sense of self. "The key to recovery for individuals who display social paralysis is that they begin to take greater responsibility for their own inner authority and intuitive feelings about food choices," states Kaminski. "By coming to a greater sense of their own self-worth and wisdom, they will make food choices that are nurturing, positive, and life fulfilling.

The key flower essences to facilitate this are Goldenrod, Pine, Cerato, Quaking Grass, Buttercup, Walnut, Joshua Tree, Mariposa Lily, Baby Blue Eyes, Rock Water, Purple Monkeyflower, and Self-Heal.

Stress and Strain: "This eating syndrome is particularly endemic to modern society and probably affects all individuals to some degree," observes Kaminski. In this pattern, the person lacks human warmth and community around eating and exerts little care in preparing and partaking of food. Eating on the run and relying on fast-food is the typical pattern. The soul longs for the qualities of sacredness, respect, gratitude, and social sharing. "Rather than fighting against the rhythm of time, such an individual needs to learn to breathe with positive aspects of time and human living, emphasizing soulful and artistic pleasure and interest in the preparation and the eating of food."

Indicated flower essences are Impatiens, Dill, Morning Glory,

Quaking Grass, Zinnia, Dandelion, Rosemary, Scleranthus, Indian Pink, Rabbitbrush, Lavender, Self-Heal, Star Tulip, Hound's Tongue, California Pitcher Plant, California Wild Rose, Shooting Star, Nasturtium, Sweet Pea, and Five-Flower Formula.

Gambling

Kaminski pairs gambling and shoplifting as similar addictions, whereas a shopping addiction is in a different category. "In shoplifting and gambling, it's the adrenal rush. It's the risk. If you talk to gambling addicts, they will tell you that they know rationally they shouldn't do it, but the thrill of the moment, the high that comes over them when everything is at stake, is hard to resist."

She likens the thrill to that reported by people who engage in extreme sports. "It's interesting that a lot of sports people are gamblers," she notes. "This is not only because it's easy to get into gambling when you're involved in sports (there's a lot of betting), but also because of what I call a Mars archetype—to risk everything and to feel that adrenal rush for a while." (Mars, associated with the Greek Ares, was the god of war in the Roman pantheon. Astrologically, the planet Mars is associated with desire, energy, and action.) For example, one man with a gambling addiction who came to Kaminski for help had been a jockey when he was younger. When the thrill of the horse race and crossing the finish line was no longer accessible to him, he turned to gambling.

What the soul needs in the case of gambling addiction is for the individual "to find ways to be courageous in life, to learn how to take risks in areas where they can do so legitimately, rather than bankrupting themselves and their families."

Although denial is a component in all forms of addiction, it is especially strong in gambling addiction, Kaminski notes, adding that this addiction is much harder to treat than others. "Gamblers are particularly adept at hiding their addiction." For this, the flower essence Black-Eyed Susan is useful, as it helps people to see their shadow side. This is the part that contains all they dislike and deny in themselves, the part they have repressed and kept hidden even from their own awareness. As they begin to reconstruct their lives and search for ways to take meaningful risks, a number of remedies support this process. One is Mountain Pride, which helps one "to be a warrior and find places where being a warrior is good," says Kaminski.

Shopping

Shopping addiction, which as noted above is a different kind of addiction from shoplifting, is an attempt to fill a hole, an emptiness inside. The soul's longing is for wholeness, Kaminski says. Buying something gives addicts a momentary sensation of wholeness, but as with other addictions, the sensation doesn't last and they need another fix.

"Of course, shopping addiction is one of those addictions that's also cultural," she observes. "It's a miasm in the whole culture. We are all trained almost from day one that we're going to be happier if we have more things. This means that in treating the addiction, you're not only dealing with that person as an individual, you're dealing with the whole culture."

A common flower essence for this type of addiction is Sagebrush. "We actually want to help the person feel okay with emptiness. This is the classic Zen state of consciousness—to have zero and for zero to be everything, the sense of spaciousness that comes of having nothing." In addition to taking this remedy, it is important to deal with the addiction in behavioral ways, she states. For this, she focuses on helping the person to learn to give away rather than accumulate, to learn to simplify, which Sagebrush also facilitates.

Stimulating Consciousness

Kaminski cautions against approaching flower essence therapy in a similar mode to "using," merely substituting a natural, safe product for harmful substances and behaviors. To regard flower essences as the "magic bullet" that will fix addiction is to misunderstand the true nature of healing. Flower essence therapy, like many other forms of natural medicine, works on the layers of a person and is a process, not a quick fix, says Kaminski. "It's a developmental process for the soul. The developmental process involves steps, metamorphoses that have to happen. We have to work in a way to bring the consciousness up in the person. Whereas in typical medicine, what we do is mask the consciousness, what we do with flower essences is try to stimulate the consciousness to see these pictures, these parts of the soul."

In summary, "flower essences help people deal with the things they need to deal with in order to move on with their lives," she states. The following cases illustrate this and the profound role that flower essences can play in reversing addiction.

Francie: The Secrets Hidden in Food Addiction

Francie, 34, was five feet, five inches in height and weighed 170 pounds. She had struggled with her weight all her life, but until three years before she came to Kaminski, it had been a cycle of gaining five to ten pounds and then losing it, albeit with difficulty. But then she became unable to control her eating and began piling on the weight, which reached 180 pounds at one point. Around this time Francie had started thinking about having children. She felt she couldn't because her body was in no shape to handle pregnancy and childbirth.

While her weight problem was of great concern to her, it was her behavior around eating that finally drove her to seek help. She was unable to resist eating sweets. If she opened a package of cookies, she couldn't leave the package alone. If she ate one, she had to eat them all. If there was a container of ice cream in the freezer, she couldn't get the thought of it out of her mind. And once she had one bite, she would eat the whole thing. When she reported all this to Kaminski at their first meeting, she also relayed that she didn't get any pleasure from this eating. Kaminski notes that she typically sees this driven quality in those with a food addiction.

Francie was always on diets, vowing to be strict with herself and eat only grapefruits or whatever the latest fad diet dictated. Once, she went on a fast and then broke it by eating a half-gallon of ice cream.

At the time that her weight ballooned out of control, she had begun eating in secret. She would sneak food into the house and hide it, telling herself that she wasn't going to eat it. While informing friends and family that she was on a diet, she would hide the "forbidden foods" in a closet and secretly consume her stashes. She also started taking a lot of laxatives and giving herself enemas and tried several times to throw up after she ate. Although she was unsuccessful at inducing vomiting, she felt she was heading in the direction of bulimia and was worried. In addition, the diet roller coaster and the abuse of laxatives had caused problems in Francie's digestion and intestines. Intestinal pain, bloating, and constipation alternating with diarrhea were chronic conditions for her.

Shortly before coming to Kaminski, she began to engage in a behavior that signaled to her how completely out of control she was. She would go to the supermarket and buy all the foods she was craving, then park her car where no one could see her, devour everything, and then dispose of the packages and containers before she went home so no one would know. One day, in the midst of one of these binges, she suddenly realized, "This is sick." She knew she had to get help.

In the first session with Francie, Kaminski learned that, in addition to the above patterns in regard to eating, Francie ate at odd hours, typically in the afternoon and evening. In the morning, she was never hungry. That's when she resolved to stay on her diet and be "good" that day. "She was always trying to model to her friends that she was 'good,'" recalls Kaminski. "At work, she would often say, 'For lunch today I'm going to have a Diet Coke and a low-cal burger without the bun.' Then on the way home, she would stop off and have some doughnuts. There was this good girl, bad girl thing. Good girl is the public display. Bad girl is secret, and no one sees her. This was a major part of her emotional picture."

The first flower essence formula Kaminski used with Francie contained Morning Glory, Manzanita, and Self-Heal, which worked synergistically, each enhancing the effects of the others.

The Morning Glory was to help stabilize Francie's life rhythms, including her eating rhythms, which is vital with any substance abuse. "People who are addicted have totally lost connection with the metabolic rhythms in the body," Kaminski explains. "Metabolically, we should eat our most nutritiously dense meal in the morning. What I've seen over and over again with people who have eating addictions, and other substance abuse too, especially cocaine or any stimulants, is that they're not hungry in the morning and they have this nighttime persona of one kind or another."

In working with addiction cases, Kaminski sets up a strict schedule for clients to take the remedies, which itself contributes to restoring the life rhythm. In Francie's case, she took her flower essence formula three times a day at set times. This approach also helps rebuild the will, which in addiction is "nearly paralyzed" as a result of repeatedly intending to follow through on a resolve and being unable to do so. The regimen for taking the remedies provides small steps toward "regaining a sense of mastery of the will." As further assistance in restoring the life rhythm and the will, Kaminski urged Francie to eat in the morning even if she didn't feel hungry.

Manzanita, which Kaminski often uses in cases of addiction, is indicated for "people who have a strong love/hate relationship with their body. They indulge in some way and at the same time they loathe their bodies." Francie had said, "I feel like I'm two people; I'm constantly warring with myself," which was an indicator of a need for this flower essence. Manzanita promotes bodily awareness, the knowledge of the body as sacred, and the capacity to nurture the body and feel the joy of being in a physical form.

The third flower essence in Francie's formula was Self-Heal, which is "a foundational remedy that could probably be used in almost every flower essence case," says Kaminski. "It helps people to feel they are in charge of their healing, that instead of being victims they can make decisions to turn their health around. It awakens the part of the body that knows how to heal itself. If we can call upon the innate wisdom of the body and let it work, the body will start to go in a self-healing direction."

Self-Heal is also important when working with addiction because it helps prevent the problem of simply replacing one substance with another, in which case healing can't occur. Self-Heal keeps the healing centered where it needs to be—within.

In the first two months of taking this formula, there were not many outward changes, but Francie became aware of just how much she hated her body and how the eating and the laxatives were a "self-violence," as she phrased it.

In the third month, after this awareness had surfaced, Kaminski gave her the flower essences Crab Apple and Hound's Tongue. Crab Apple works on revulsion for the body, especially when it is accompanied by hyper-attention to cleansing, as evidenced in Francie's case by the overuse of laxatives and enemas. Francie's body type indicated Hound's Tongue. From her chest up, she didn't look overweight. She carried all her weight in the lower portion of her body. This reflected back to her statement about the two warring parts of her. "It was like one part didn't want to be here and the other part was entrenched and pulled down by gravity," observes Kaminski.

The hound's tongue plant resembles Francie's physical form in that it has large basal leaves that lie on the ground and it sends up celestial blue flowers. "All plants have some kind of polarity. We give certain flower essences to help that polarity resolve itself in a human being." In Francie's case, she had a lot of security issues and material concerns, about money, advancing in her job, worry over the future. She hung on too tightly to anything that gave her a sense of grounding, so she resembled the hound's tongue plant emotionally as well as physically.

Francie continued taking the original formula along with the two additional remedies. While Francie felt better on this regimen, Kaminski began to feel that for Francie to reach resolution on her food addiction, something more had to happen. At that point, she asked her to start keeping a food diary, which she now does automatically when working with anybody who has food issues. Francie was one of her early cases.

In the diary, Francie described an event that occurred one Saturday night when friends were coming for dinner and there was a carton of ice cream in the freezer for their dessert. She had been sticking to her diet and told herself that the ice cream was for the evening meal and she was not going to open it before then. She remembers walking into the kitchen and then everything went blank. When she "came to," she had eaten the whole carton of ice cream. "I hated myself. But I couldn't account for that time. I was not unconscious, but it was like I was in a trance. During that time, I wasn't there."

"With alcoholism, we say people black out. That's a more physiological blackout," states Kaminski. "But with addiction, whether it's sex addiction or food addiction or whatever, there are emotional blackouts all the time. It's as though another part of the self completely takes over. The higher self goes dormant or is subsumed, and this other sub-personality says, 'I'm driving the car now. Get out of the way.'"

Upon hearing Francie's story, Kaminski had Francie stop taking the other flower essences and started her on Black-Eyed Susan alone. As noted earlier, this flower essence helps bring the shadow side of a person into the light. "I realized that what we had to get to was her consciously confronting this part of herself that had another agenda."

From that point, outward changes began to occur. Francie stopped bingeing for the most part and started steadily losing weight. Then the issue underlying her food addiction emerged.

Francie had grown up in Los Angeles in a wealthy family. Her mother was beautiful and emotionally distant. Francie idolized her from a distance. She remembers her parents always dressed up and going out, very much a part of the elite social scene. She was left in the care of a nanny who was quite overweight. The nanny gave her the love that her mother didn't. Francie felt both a revulsion and a deep love for this woman.

"If we work long enough with any addiction, we usually come to some kind of core concept from the culture, the religion, the family system—and it is different in every person." In Francie's case, there was a polarity of "the solid grounding, the love, the nurturance on one side, and on the other, beauty, but it was cold, unavailable, and unattainable."

Based on this background, Kaminski had the insight to take Francie to another level through the flower essences Madrone, Mariposa Lily, and Chocolate Lily.

Madrone is indicated for a mixed experience of the physical world, with both revulsion and comfort in connection to the physical. It helped Francie explore the source of her revulsion. As a child, on the one side was her mother who looked like a starlet—glamorous, beautiful, with a slim body and dyed blonde hair—but was emotionally cold. She wanted her mother to love her; instead her mother constantly abandoned her. On the other side was her nanny—large, like a bowl of jelly—who was lovable and loving. "I got lost in her body when she hugged me," recalled Francie. She realized that what she felt was, "I want this, but I hate this."

"If we work long enough with any addiction, we usually come to some kind of core concept from the culture, the religion, the family system—and it is different in every person." In Francie's case, there was a polarity of "the solid grounding, the love, the nurturance on one side, and on the other, beauty, but it was cold, unavailable, and unattainable."

As for the other components of Francie's new formula, all the lilies work on the feminine principle in one form or another, explains Kaminski. Mariposa Lily, from a pure white flower that grows in alpine regions, addresses the mother wound (pain and trauma associated with one's mother). Chocolate Lily, from a dark reddish brown flower that grows in the grasslands, is often indicated when there is constriction or obstruction in the bowel, and also in cases of endometriosis. These two flower essences addressed the two polarities of mothering that Francie experienced and helped unite the warring aspects of her soul.

Kaminski cautions that it is essential for the flower essence therapist to be there as a counselor for the client as the flower essences stir up archetypes and uncover issues in the soul that have been buried. Emotional support when difficult feelings begin surfacing is a vital part of the healing process.

As it happened, Francie's mother, who Francie had learned was an alcoholic, was very ill with liver cancer and getting chemotherapy at the time that Francie began to do her deeper healing. Francie felt unable to love her despite her failing condition. On a visit to her mother after she began taking the Madrone, Mariposa Lily, and Chocolate Lily, however, she was able to hug her. She felt revulsion, but also love for the first time. "Her dying mother became an opportunity for her to heal her deep soul issue," observes Kaminski.

As for Francie's food addiction, the bingeing had turned around in the first four months of flower essence therapy, and she now felt in control of her eating. Occasionally, she would report that she had "pigged out," but it happened less and less, and when it did, she felt it was a conscious choice.

Another change was in her enjoyment of food. When she indulged and ate a chocolate bar now, she truly enjoyed it. The result was that she didn't need to indulge as often. "When we start to enjoy, to take pleasure in our food, we need less of it," says Kaminski. Eating breakfast, a higher protein diet, and complex carbohydrates instead of simple carbohydrates also helped restore Francie's metabolic balance, which contributed to her natural move toward health.

Francie had already begun losing poundage before she uncovered the emotional issues, but delving into them was what finally stabilized her weight. She got down to 140 pounds, which she felt was a good weight for her, and that was where she stayed.

"Toward the end of our work together, which lasted for 13 months, her mother died, and that was a major transition for her," recalls Kaminski. "She was able to have a deep emotional connection with her mother before she died, really help her, and cry and express her grief. That was powerful." Kaminski credits the flower essences with helping Francie to be able to do that.

Two and a half years later, Francie got pregnant. Stabilizing her weight and relationship to food and working on her unresolved mother issues freed her to become a mother herself.

Jeremy: Leaving Marijuana

Jeremy, 29, lived in a big marijuana-growing area. He sought Kaminski's help after a friend of his was arrested for selling. It had scared Jeremy because he said it could just as easily have been him. This came after another incident in which someone in his circle of acquaintances used a gun in an attempt to steal some marijuana, and a police investigation was under way. This brought home to Jeremy that he was in a bad crowd and going nowhere.

He supported himself by selling marijuana and doing the odd carpentry or construction job when money was tight. He also occasionally sang and played backup in a band, but his musical abilities were only average, neither bad nor particularly good. He felt that was the theme of his life, telling Kaminski, "I have a lot of talent, but nothing is developed very well, and I'm not moving."

He had begun smoking marijuana in his teens, and his use had escalated over the years. Now he smoked every day, beginning in the morning. Whenever he didn't smoke, he felt apprehensive and ill at ease. When he did smoke, he felt paranoid, and one of his primary fears was of getting arrested. His smoking was partly a social activity. In his crowd, that's what everybody did when they got together, he said.

Another event that set him thinking that he needed to make a change was that he had been in an on-again, off-again relationship with a woman who had finally broken away from him and their social circle a few months earlier. She was younger than he, in her mid-twenties, and had decided to go back to school. When she ended their relationship, she told him, "I'm finished being a kid. Now it's time for me to grow up and do something with my life."

It was a wake-up call for him that she didn't want to be involved with him or their crowd anymore because she wanted to make something of her life. She wasn't the only one. Jeremy had been noticing that friends from high school were moving to different places, accomplishing things, manifesting their dreams. Meanwhile the crowd he was hanging out with "was becoming more and more degenerate." He told Kaminski, "I'm just drifting into this place that I never wanted to be, but I don't know how to get out of it." Recognizing that is what brought him to treatment. He wanted to stop smoking marijuana so much and was having trouble doing it on his own.

As with Francie, Kaminski started with three flower essences. Again, Morning Glory was a basic one to help stabilize the life rhythms skewed by an addictive lifestyle. California Poppy, which is commonly used for the psychotropic (of substances that act on the mind) addictions, was another key remedy for Jeremy.

She notes that this is the state flower of California, which to her is appropriate because "in a way, California is the land of delusional seeking. There are plenty of good things in our culture, but there is this capacity always to want the easy life. The California Poppy flower essence can help move a person out of wanting the easy path, wanting the path of instant enlightenment, instant light, or feeling good right now." The path of enlightenment is what the soul is craving in marijuana addiction. The drug may make you think you are getting that, but you are not as long as you are using a drug to get there, says Kaminski. The result is that the soul's longing is not met.

The third flower essence in Jeremy's formula was Agrimony, which facilitates "taking off the mask." Kaminski notes that "being perceived as 'cool' and 'in control' is part of a persona in which many individuals who use drugs in social situations are invested." Healing requires removing the mask of that persona.

After starting Jeremy on these remedies, Kaminski began to explore with him what he wanted to do in life. He said that he had always wanted to be an artist. His teachers had told him that he had talent. In fact, he still sculpted and painted some, but like the music, he didn't fully apply himself. It was the same with the carpentry that he did for occasional money.

As part of this exploration of life goals, Kaminski asked him what he was going to replace marijuana with. "It's not a matter of just stopping the addiction," she emphasizes. "With an addiction like his, you have to find out what is going to replace whole parts of his life. There's a full-fledged lifestyle that has to be addressed." In Jeremy's case, his real self hadn't emerged, though he was 29. "He hadn't found the right relationship, the right goals in his life. He seemed lost. That's another way that addiction works. It replaces who you are and what your real life goals are."

In answer to what he was going to do instead of hanging out and smoking marijuana, Jeremy said he would like to go to art school, but he didn't have any money. He decided to commit to carpentry and work every day instead of doing odd jobs now and then, so he could save money. He followed through on this plan and stopped selling marijuana. He also moved into town into a new environment. His efforts to quit smoking weren't successful until he made this move. He had to get away from the social scene in which smoking marijuana was a central activity.

Two months after Jeremy started flower essence treatment, Kaminski changed his formula to a combination of California Poppy, Wild Oat, Blackberry, and Goldenrod. Wild Oat is a classic remedy to give to young people around 27 or 28 years old, she explains, when the burning questions are: "What is my life's destiny? What am I here to do? Am I just going to sow wild oats all my life, or am I going to hear who I really am? Am I going to listen to my calling in life, my vocation?" Blackberry facilitates "the focus and engagement of the will toward practical tasks and manifestation on Earth."

Kaminski and other flower essence therapists often give Goldenrod to young people who use drugs because their drug use is typically due to their social scene. Goldenrod carries the message, "My identity is not only horizontal but vertical." It supports "the vertical integration of the personality so that it feels its aloneness in a healthy way." This and the Wild Oat would help Jeremy know that "his identity was not based on what his friends were doing, that he stood in his own strength, integrity, and aloneness—aloneness in the good sense of the word."

Jeremy worked with Kaminski for eight months. In the fourth month, he began to delve deeper in their sessions. He revealed that his father had left his mother when Jeremy was a year old and had not been in touch with the family since. His mother was in two other relationships while he was growing up, each of which produced a sister for him. They moved around and lived in "trashed-out" homes, Jeremy relayed, and there were nights that his mother didn't come home. He was like a father to his younger sisters, making them breakfast and attending to them in his mother's absence. Jeremy was home-schooled for a while, but not very well. He began to see that no one had ever given him structure and it was needed in his present life. He realized that while he didn't get it in his childhood, he could set it up for himself now.

Jeremy began to feel the need to make contact with his father. At that point, in addition to the California Poppy and the Goldenrod, Kaminski gave him Baby Blue Eyes and Sunflower to help heal "the wounded masculine." Baby Blue Eyes is the corollary to Mariposa Lily (which helps heal the mother wound), addressing "wounding from the father, for men or women whose father wasn't there." Sunflower provides solar radiance that asks, "How can I shine? How can I be positive?"

Jeremy tracked down his father and summoned the courage to call him. His father didn't want to talk to him, which was heartbreaking, but Jeremy wasn't sorry that he had made the call. It had been important for him to do that in order to move forward in his life.

During his eight months of flower essence therapy, when things were really difficult for Jeremy, he would smoke, but it happened less and less as time went on. When he initially stopped smoking, he said,

"I feel a hole in my soul," which he realized was what marijuana had filled for him. When he felt the hole, he took his flower essences a little more frequently. Gradually, the empty feeling subsided.

Jeremy, who had begun sculpting more, decided to relocate to a city in another state, where there was an art program he was interested in. The last flower essence formula Kaminski gave him before he left was one to encourage strength. It contained Sunflower, Goldenrod, Wild Oat, and Larch. "These were all positive masculine remedies to help him move out into the world, to develop his talent," she explains. Larch supports the development of confidence, especially for men. "It helps activate the archetype that fathers should ideally model for their sons."

Jeremy kept in touch for a while after his move, reporting that he was involved with a community program devoted to doing art with inner-city children. He continued with his sculpture, showing several pieces in an art gallery and selling a few as well. The last Kaminski heard from him, he was going to school so he could work as a counselor. He had found through providing emotional support to the children in the art program that he liked that work even more than art.

7 The Five Levels of Healing

While many people speak generally of the body-mind-spirit connection, Dietrich Klinghardt, M.D., Ph.D., based in Bellevue, Washington, has developed a detailed model that explains that connection in terms of Five Levels of Healing: the Physical Level, the Electromagnetic Level, the Mental Level, the Intuitive Level, and the Spiritual Level. The model provides a comprehensive way to understand and approach the treatment of any illness, including addiction.

Dr. Klinghardt is internationally acclaimed for this brilliant model of healing and for developing a number of therapeutic techniques (see "About the Therapies and Techniques" at the end of this chapter) that have proven useful in the treatment of a broad range of conditions. He trains doctors around the world in both his model and in the use of the therapies he developed.

Health and illness are a reflection of the state of the five levels in a given individual. Addiction, like any health problem, can originate on any of the levels. A basic principle of Dr. Klinghardt's paradigm is that an interference or imbalance on one level, if untreated, spreads upward or downward to the other levels. Thus, addiction can involve multiple levels, sometimes even all five, if the originating imbalance was not correctly addressed. Each of the factors discussed in chapter 2 falls on one or sometimes two of the five levels. For example, nutritional deficiencies exert their effects on the Physical Level, while heavy metal toxicity creates interference on both the Physical and Electromagnetic levels.

Another basic principle is that healing interventions can be implemented at any of the levels. Unless upper-level imbalances are addressed, restoring balance at the lower levels will not produce long-lasting effects. Thus, treating only the biochemistry of addiction may not resolve the problem for some people. Biochemical therapies only address the Physical Level of illness and healing and leave the causes at the Intuitive Level, for example, intact. The corrected factors will soon be thrown off again by the downward cascade of this imbalance.

The Five Levels of Healing model also provides a useful framework for the natural medicine therapies covered in this book. They each approach addiction by identifying and treating disturbances at the different levels. In keeping with the holism of natural medicine, a number of the therapeutic modalities function on several levels. For example, traditional Chinese medicine (chapter 5) works on both the Physical and the Electromagnetic Levels, while Matrix therapy (chapter 8) works on the Electromagnetic and Mental Levels (see the sidebar "Natural Medicine and the Five Levels of Healing," p. 153).

The following sections describe the Five Levels of Healing, discuss how they interact with addiction, and identify therapies that can remove interference at each level. Keep in mind that interference at different levels can manifest as the same condition in different people, so while the source of the problem for one person with a cocaine addiction, for example, may be on the first level, the source may be on the fourth level for another person with the same type of addiction.

The First Level: The Physical Body

The Physical Body includes all the functions on the physical plane, such as the structure and biochemistry of the body. Interference or imbalance at this level can result from an injury or anything that alters the structure, such as accidents, concussions, dental work, or surgery. "Surgery modulates the structure by creating scars or adhesions in the bones and ligaments, which changes the way things act on the Physical Level," says Dr. Klinghardt.

Imbalance at the first level can also result from anything that alters the biochemistry such as poor diet, too much or too little of a nutrient in the diet or in nutritional supplements, or taking the wrong supplements for one's particular biochemistry. Organisms such as bacteria, viruses, and parasites can also change the host's biochemistry. "They all take over the host to some degree and change the host's behavior by modulating its biochemistry," Dr. Klinghardt explains.

"The whole world of toxicity also belongs in the field of biochemistry," he says. Toxic elements that can alter biochemistry include heavy metals such as mercury, insecticides, pesticides, and other environmental chemicals. Interestingly, heavy metals operate on both the Physical Level and the next level of healing, the Electromagnetic Level. Due to their metallic nature, they can alter the biochemistry by creating electromagnetic disturbances. Research has also found a connection between mercury toxicity and addiction. "Several studies have shown that mercury in the brain causes addictive cravings," notes Dr. Klinghardt.

Interference at the Physical Level can result in a wide range of disorders, including symptoms of mental illness and problems with addiction, he says. A common factor in addiction is nutritional deficiencies—of amino acids, for instance. Dr. Klinghardt cites the efficacy of programs that stabilize the amino acids in stopping alcoholic and drug cravings. In most cases, he believes that this is a symptomatic fix because in his experience the cause of addiction is usually found at the fourth or fifth level. "But the symptomatic fix is certainly better than drinking or doing drugs," he notes.

The therapeutic modalities that function at this level are those that address biochemical or structural aspects, from nutritional supplements, herbal medicine, and hormone therapy to mechanical therapies such as chiropractic.

 For more about amino acids, see chapter 3. For more about other nutritional deficiencies, see chapter 2.

The Second Level: The Electromagnetic Body

The Electromagnetic Body is the body's energetic field. Dr. Klinghardt explains it in terms of the traffic of information in the nervous system. "Eighty percent of the messages go up to the brain [from the body], and 20 percent of the messages go down from the brain [to the body]. The nerve currents moving up and down generate a magnetic field that goes out into space, creating an electromagnetic field around the body that interacts with other fields." Acupuncture meridians (energy channels) and the chakra system are part of the Electromagnetic Body.

A *chakra,* which means "wheel" in Sanskrit, is an energy vortex or center in the nonphysical counterpart (energy field) of the body. There are seven major chakras positioned roughly from the base of the spine, with points along the spine, to the crown of the head. As with acupuncture meridians, when chakras are blocked, the free flow of energy in the body's field is impeded. While Hindu in origin, the concept of chakras is gaining attention in the West in both therapeutic and spiritual applications.

 For more about chakras, see chapter 8.

Biophysical stress is a source of disturbance at the Electromagnetic Level. Biophysical stress is electromagnetic interference from devices that have their own electromagnetic fields, such as electric wall outlets, televisions, microwaves, cell phones, cell phone towers, power lines, and radio stations. These interfere with the electromagnetic system in and around the body.

For example, if you sleep with your head near an electric outlet in the wall, the electromagnetic field from that outlet interferes with your own. An outlet may not even have to be involved. Simply sleeping with your head near a wall in which electric cables run can be sufficient to throw your field off. The brain's blood vessels typically contract in response to the man-made electromagnetic field, leading to decreased blood flow in the brain, says Dr. Klinghardt. Repositioning your bed can remedy this interference.

Geopathic stress, or electromagnetic emissions from the Earth, is another source of disturbance. Underground streams and fault lines are a source of these emissions. Again, proximity of your bed to one of these sources—for example, directly over a fault line—can throw your own electromagnetic field out of balance and produce a wide range of symptoms, notes Dr. Klinghardt. The remedy may again be as simple as shifting the position of your bed in the room.

Interference at the second level can cascade down to the Physical Level. The constriction of the blood vessels in the brain in response to biophysical or geopathic stress results in the blood carrying less oxygen and nutrients to the brain, explains Dr. Klinghardt. The ensuing deficiencies are a biochemical disturbance, with obvious implications for brain function and mental health. If such deficiencies have their root at the Electromagnetic Level, however, it is important to know that you cannot fix them by taking certain supplements to correct the biochemistry, he cautions.

For example, if an individual has a zinc deficiency, supplementing with zinc may correct the problem if it is merely a biochemical disturbance (a first-level issue). If the restriction of blood flow in the brain as a result of sleeping too close to an electrical outlet (a second-level issue) is behind the deficiency, taking zinc may seem to resolve the problem, but it will return when the person stops taking the supplement. Moving the bed away from the outlet will stop the electromagnetic interference and prevent the recurrence of a zinc deficiency.

Physical trauma or scars can also throw off the second level. "If a scar crosses an acupuncture meridian, it completely alters the energy flow in the system," observes Dr. Klinghardt. An infected tooth or a root canal can accomplish the same. Neural Therapy (which involves the injection of local anesthetics such as procaine or natural healing substances into specific sites in the body to clear interferences in the flow of electrical energy and restore proper nerve function) can remove the energetic disturbance created by scars and injuries. Biological dentistry (which uses only nontoxic dental materials and recognizes the relationship between dental factors and overall health) can remedy dental interferences.

Heavy metal toxicity, from mercury dental fillings and/or environmental metals in the air, water, and food supply, can block the entire electromagnetic system. "We know that the ganglia can be disturbed by a number of things, but toxicity in general is often responsible for throwing off the electromagnetic impulses." (Ganglia are nerve bundles that are like relay stations for nerve impulses.)

Mercury and other heavy metals produce disturbances on both

the Physical and Electromagnetic Levels. The leaching of mercury from fillings is an ongoing source of exposure to a known neurotoxin, which is a Physical Level factor, but "probably the more important effect in terms of mental illness is that each metal has a strong electromagnetic field around it," notes Dr. Klinghardt. "The upper teeth are close to the brain. The electromagnetic field of metal crowns, metal fillings, and metal bridges impairs the blood flow inside the brain, and that's a very important thing with all mental illnesses," which is the category in which addiction is placed. As noted previously, research has found a link between the presence of mercury in the body and addictive cravings.

In addition to the role mercury plays in addiction, substance abuse is one way that the body attempts to deal with the energy disturbance caused by heavy metals. Eliminating exposure and undergoing detoxification may be important steps in correcting the energy imbalance and removing the impetus toward addiction.

A combination of biophysical or geopathic stress and heavy metal toxicity is particularly problematic. Heavy metals are found mostly in the brain, where they work like antennae, says Dr. Klinghardt. They pick up the electromagnetic or geopathic interference, exacerbating the disturbance to a person's energy field and worsening associated symptoms and conditions.

In addition to the role mercury plays in addiction, substance abuse is one way that the body attempts to deal with the energy disturbance caused by heavy metals. Eliminating exposure and undergoing detoxification may be important steps in correcting the energy imbalance and removing the impetus toward addiction.

It may not be necessary to have your mercury fillings taken out, however. In fact, if removal is not done correctly, it can be more harmful than leaving the fillings in, Dr. Klinghardt cautions. Removal needs to be done by a dentist who has been trained in how to do it safely and effectively, as mercury vapors and particles are released during the removal process. In addition, a detoxification protocol needs to be implemented after the fillings have been replaced with non-mercury composite fillings.

 For information about dental mercury, see the websites of: Dr. Joseph Mercola at www.mercola.com and Dental Amalgam Mercury Syndrome (DAMS) at www.dams.cc. For help in locating a dentist, call the DAMS National Office at 800-311-6265.

A person's level of mercury and other heavy metal toxicity can be measured through hair analysis, which shows the levels of minerals and heavy metals in the body. For a more precise heavy metal analysis, Dr. Klinghardt uses an injection of a chelating agent (DMPS), which binds with heavy metals and carries them out of the body in the urine (see Chelation in "About the Therapies and Techniques"). A subsequent check of the urine reveals which toxic metals are present. In his practice, patients with substance abuse problems typically test high for heavy metals. To get the metals out of the body, he relies on oral chelation, using known natural chelators such as cilantro and chlorella that can be taken as oral supplements. He sometimes uses intravenous chelation (which requires the insertion of a needle into a vein to deliver the chelating substances slowly via an IV drip) with the amino acid glutathione, which is more aggressive in getting metals out of the brain.

Allergies, like heavy metals, create interference on both the Physical and Electromagnetic levels and are a common factor in addiction. Chronic allergic reaction keeps the immune system in an activated state, which weakens immunity (Physical), and the presence of allergenic substances disturbs the body's energy field (Electromagnetic). "When you're allergic to something, there are two outcomes: you are miserable when you take or are exposed to the allergen, or you become addicted to it." Dr. Klinghardt observes that the latter is frequently the case in addiction, as discussed in chapter 4. "Often people are allergic to something in the drug they use, and that makes them crave it. It is an odd twist in the brain that the things you're allergic to you often crave."

To eliminate allergies, Dr. Klinghardt uses a form of NAET (see

"About the Therapies and Techniques" and chapter 4). "What you're doing with this in terms of addiction is basically stabilizing the system," he says. "Eliminating allergies to the substance the person craves very quickly cuts down the craving."

In addition to the techniques discussed above, traditional acupuncture is a primary therapy for the second level of healing, as it removes electromagnetic interference and restores the proper energy flow in the body.

 For more about allergies and NAET, see chapter 4. For more on acupuncture, see chapter 5.

The Third Level: The Mental Body

The third level is the Mental Level or the Mental Body, also known as the Thought Field. This is where your attitudes, beliefs, and early childhood experiences reside. "This is the home of psychology," says Dr. Klinghardt. He explains that the Mental Body is outside the Physical Body, rather than housed in the brain. "Memory, thinking, and the mind are all phenomena outside the Physical Body; they are not happening in the brain. The Mental Body is an energetic field."

Disturbances at this level come from traumatic experiences, which can begin as early as conception. Early trauma, or an unresolved conflict situation, leaves faulty circuitry in the Mental Body, explains Dr. Klinghardt. For example, if at two years old, your parents divorced and your father was not allowed by law to see you, you may have formed the beliefs that your father didn't love you and that it was your fault your parents broke up because you are inherently bad. These damaging beliefs are faulty mental circuitry.

The mind replays traumatic experiences over and over, keeping constant stress signals running through the autonomic nervous system. These disturbances trickle down and affect the Electromagnetic Level of healing, changing nerve function by triggering the constriction of blood vessels and, in turn, affecting the biochemical level in the form of nutritional deficiency.

It may look like a biochemical disturbance, says Dr. Klinghardt, but the cause is much higher up. "Again, this is a situation you cannot treat with lasting results by giving someone supplements or acupuncture." You have to address the third-level interference, the problem in the Mental Body.

Despite what people may conclude from the related names, so-called mental disorders—now more popularly termed "brain disorders," of which addiction is one—aren't necessarily a function of disturbance in the Mental Body. The cause can be on any of the five levels of healing, iterates Dr. Klinghardt. In his experience, in most cases of addiction, the third level is not the source. "It's more the fourth and fifth levels, and sometimes the first level."

One primary exception is prescription drug abuse, which is typically a third-level issue, he says. "I find that this has a different character from other addictions. In this, people tend to be self-medicating posttraumatic stress disorder, which they have from their childhood or early years."

One of the therapies Dr. Klinghardt uses to address disturbances at this level is Thought Field Therapy or TFT (see "About the Therapies and Techniques"), which actually operates on the boundary between the second and third levels. Unlike psychotherapy, another method that works on this level but which is an extended undertaking, TFT works quickly to clear trauma in many cases.

"A large number of addictions respond to Thought Field Therapy, from cigarette smoking all the way up to heroin addiction," says Dr. Klinghardt. He has found that tobacco addiction is particularly responsive to TFT. Both heavy metal toxicity and allergies can prevent it from working, however. While the treatment may produce relief at first, it will not hold as it does with people for whom these factors are not an issue—a fact that supports the need to clear toxicity and allergies.

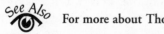 **For more about Thought Field Therapy, see chapter 8.**

In addition to Thought Field Therapy, to effect healing at the third level Dr. Klinghardt uses a method he developed called Applied Psychoneurobiology (see "About the Therapies and Techniques"), which is also useful at the fourth level. Among the other therapeutic modalities that work at the Mental Level are hypnotherapy and homeopathy.

The Fourth Level: The Intuitive Body

The fourth level is the Intuitive Body. Some people call it the Dream Body. Experience on this level includes dream states, trance states, and ecstasy, as well as states with a negative association such as nightmares, possession, and curses. The Intuitive Body is what Swiss depth psychologist C. G. Jung called the collective unconscious. "On the fourth level, humans are deeply connected with each other and also with flora, fauna, and the global environment," says Dr. Klinghardt.

In his experience, the fourth level is the most common in addiction. "You usually have to go to the fourth level to learn why people are doing this self-destructive behavior. If the source is at this level and you don't address it, you have no chance with any of the other techniques. Nothing will work." Given this, with people who come to Dr. Klinghardt for help in overcoming their addictions, he usually goes straight to the fourth level. Clearing that level and using Thought Field Therapy to take care of any residual interference at the second/third level are very often all that is needed. "We have a dramatic success rate with that approach," he states.

Interference at this level comes from a previous generation in the family. "The cause and effect are separated by several generations. It goes over time and space," explains Dr. Klinghardt. Rather than a genetic inheritance of a physical weakness, it is an energetic legacy of an injustice with which the family never dealt. It can manifest as almost any physical or mental illness.

The range of specific issues that can be the source is vast, but it usually involves a family member who was excluded in a previous generation. When the other family members don't go through the deep process of grieving the excluded one, whether the exclusion results from separation, death, alienation, or ostracism, the psychic interference of that exclusion is passed on.

Another common systemic factor involves identification with

victims of a forebear. "A member of the family two, three, or four generations later will atone for an injustice," without even knowing who the person involved was or what they did, explains Dr. Klinghardt. For example, a woman murders her husband and is never found out. She marries again and lives a long life. Three generations later, one of her great-grandchildren is born. To atone for the murder, the child self-sacrifices by, for example, starting to take drugs as a teenager and committing a slow suicide. Or the teenager is identifying with an excluded person, and taking drugs is a way of excluding himself.

"It's a form of self-punishment that anybody can see on the outside, but nobody understands what is wrong with this child—he had loving parents, good nutrition, went to a good school, and look what he's doing now, he's on drugs. But if you look back two or three generations, you'll see exactly why this child is self-sacrificing." Dr. Klinghardt notes that mental illness is "very often an outcome on the systemic level."

People with multiple addictions often have multiple traumas, he notes. These can be multiple traumas in their own life (a third-level factor) or multiple traumas in their family tree (a fourth-level issue). "There may have been sexual abuse on one side, murderous behavior and wars on the other side, and incest in another branch. Each of these groups causes its own addiction in the descendent. They coexist in the same person."

For healing at this level, Dr. Klinghardt uses what is known as Systemic Family Therapy, or Family Systems Therapy. This therapy involves tracing the origins of current illness back to a previous generation. For the discovery process, Dr. Klinghardt uses the form developed by German psychoanalyst Bert Hellinger. Sometimes an event is known in a family, sometimes it is not. By questioning a client, Dr. Klinghardt is usually able to discover an event from a previous generation that is a likely source of interference for the client's current condition. If no one knew about a certain event, such as the murder in the example above, there are usually clues in a family that point to those ancestors as a possible source.

For the therapy, the client or a close relative chooses audience members to represent the people in question. In our example, they would be the great-grandmother, great-grandfather, and the new husband. These people come together on a stage or central area. They are not told the story, even when the story is known. "They just go up there not knowing anything, and suddenly feel all these feelings and have all these thoughts come up. . . . Very quickly, within a minute or two, they start feeling like the real people in life have felt, or are feeling in their death now, and start interacting with each other in bizarre ways," says Dr. Klinghardt.

The client typically does not participate, but simply observes. "The therapist does careful therapeutic interventions, but there's very little needed usually." The person put up for the murdered husband stands there, with no idea of what happened in the past, but then he falls to the floor. When someone asks, "What happened to you?" he answers, "I've been murdered." It just comes out of his mouth. Then the therapist asks if he wants to say anything to any of the other people. He speaks to his wife, and it becomes clear that she was the one who murdered him. They speak back and forth, and "very quickly, there's deep healing that happens between the two," states Dr. Klinghardt. "Usually we relive the pain and the truth that was there . . . It's very, very dramatic . . . Then the therapist does some healing therapeutic intervention with those representatives."

With removal of the interference that was transmitted down the generations, the client's condition is resolved, although the trickle-down effect to the lower levels of healing may need to be addressed. Often, however, healing at the higher level is sufficient. With balance restored at that level, the other levels are then able to correct themselves.

Dr. Klinghardt likens Family Systems Therapy to shamanic work in Africa. (It could also be likened to the psychic healing discussed in chapter 9.) Shamanic healing is the ancient practice of spiritual healing used by indigenous peoples worldwide. In Africa, shamanic healing often has to be done from a distance through a representative because of the impracticability of a sick child, for example, traveling 200 miles from the village to see the medicine man. The representative holds a piece of clothing or hair from that child, and the shaman does the healing work on the stranger. "There's a magical effect broadcast back to the child," says Dr. Klinghardt. "The child often gets well. It's the same principle with Family Systems Therapy. We call it surrogate healing." He adds that this form of therapy has become very popular in Europe in the last few years, while it is still relatively new in the United States.

Dr. Klinghardt also uses Applied Psychoneurobiology (APN), the method he developed for the process of discovery and resolution of the family systems issues, which enables the work to happen with just a practitioner and the patient in a regular treatment room, accomplishing the same end without representatives of the antecedents. It uses Autonomic Response Testing (ART; see "About the Therapies and Techniques") to pinpoint what happened and engage in the dialogues that arise in this work.

He gives the example of a 45-year-old woman who had lived daily with asthma since she was two years old. Through ART, in a kind of process of elimination, Dr. Klinghardt learned that physical causes were not the source of the asthma and that it had to do with exclusion of some kind in a previous generation. Further exploration revealed that this woman had lost a younger sibling when she was two years old. In this case, the woman knew of the event, but that was all she knew. ART confirmed the connection between this buried death and the asthma. Dr. Klinghardt stopped the session at this point, instructing his client to find out what she could about this family occurrence and then come back.

The woman's mother was still alive and told her that the baby died shortly after birth, was buried behind the house without a gravestone or other marker on the site, and was never mentioned again in the family. Everyone knew where the child was buried, but there was an unspoken agreement never to speak of her. Not only that, but the

> ## In Their Own Words
>
> *"I have felt a nonspecific craving for most of my life . . . It is different from and more far-reaching than the physical craving for alcohol . . . This intense and at times painful craving is deep thirst for our own wholeness, our spiritual identity."*
>
> —Christina Grof, author and founder of the Spiritual Emergence Network, on her alcoholism[229]

149

next child born was given the same name, as if the one who had died had never existed or, worse, had been replaced.

"This was a violation of a principle of what we know about Systemic Family Therapy, which is that each member that's born into a family has the same and equal right to belong to the family." Exclusion, even in memory, is a form of injustice and creates interference energy that is transmitted through the generations. Exclusion of a family member in the past is frequently the source of disturbance at the Intuitive Level, according to Dr. Klinghardt.

The client came back for the second session, and Dr. Klinghardt put her into a light trance state. "In that trance state she was able to contact that being, the dead sibling, and say to her, 'I remember you now, I bring you back into my family, I give you a place in my heart, I will never forget you.' Then she cried, and it was a very transformative experience." He observes that this process required very little guidance from him and took only about 20 minutes.

During the session, the woman made a commitment to go back to the house where the child was buried—it was still a family property—and put a gravestone on her grave. After the session, the woman's asthma was clearly better. She rated it at 50 to 60 percent better and reported later that it stayed that way. "It took her about three months to put up the gravestone, and she said the day after she set up the gravestone for that child, her asthma disappeared completely," relates Dr. Klinghardt. That was eight years ago, and the asthma has not returned.

Dr. Klinghardt and others who practice Family Systems Therapy have seen similar connections in cases of mental illness. Addiction, chronic anxiety or depression (both of which often fuel addiction), schizophrenia, bipolar disorder, hyperactivity in children, aggressive behavior, and autism can all lead back to systemic family issues. In fact, Dr. Klinghardt estimates that "about 70 percent of mental disorders across the board go back to systemic family issues that need to be treated. People try to treat them psychologically, on the third level, and it cannot work. This is not the right level." Similarly, focusing on the biochemistry is not going to fix the problem when the source is at the fourth level.

Another therapy that operates on this level, in addition to those

---

A Smoking Legacy in Germany

Dr. Klinghardt, who is originally from Germany and sees patients there for part of each year, relates a fascinating cultural and transgenerational aspect to cigarette smoking in that country. Several studies showed that after World War II there was a huge amount of smoking going on in Germany. Then, in the next generation, very few smoked. In the second generation, the grandchildren of the smokers, the majority were smokers.

The prevailing theory traces this phenomenon back to Hitler, says Dr. Klinghardt. "It became known in the early 1930s that smoking causes lung cancer. Hitler was very scientifically oriented, and when he learned of this, he simply declared smoking un-German. Nobody in the SS or in his camp was allowed to smoke. None of those who sympathized with him smoked. The moment Hitler was dead, everybody started smoking to express their disrespect for him."

This phenomenon is now a kind of culture-wide transgenerational legacy that affects every second generation. "It's cascading down the generations," observes Dr. Klinghardt. The members of every second generation repeat their ancestors' symbolic protest, not realizing that they are smoking "to express their unconscious stand against the Nazi regime."

---

already mentioned, is transpersonal psychology. Stated simply, transpersonal refers to an acknowledgment of the phenomena of the fourth level, "the dimension where a person is affected deeply in themselves by something that isn't themselves, that is of somebody else. Transpersonal psychology is a coverup term for modern shamanism," observes Dr. Klinghardt, meaning that psychotherapists who acknowledge the importance of spiritual connection are facilitating the kind of healing that was traditionally the purview of shamans.

The Fifth Level: The Spiritual

The fifth level is the direct relationship of the patient with God, or whatever name you choose for the Divine. Interference in this relationship can be caused by early childhood experiences, past-life traumas, or enlightenment experiences with a guru or other spiritual teacher. Of the latter, Dr. Klinghardt says, "Some enlightenment experiences actually turn out to be a block. If the experience occurred in context with a guru, the person may become unable to reach there without the guru. The very thing that showed them what to look for becomes an obstacle."

Heroin addiction and alcoholism often have their source on the fifth level, says Dr. Klinghardt, "which is why the AA program works relatively well. They recognize the connection between addiction and a lack of God in the life of the person. We find that the use of heroin and alcohol is an attempt by the person to reconnect with God. That connection has been broken. Very often you have to go back into a past life or to some event that disconnected them from their trust in God."

While reestablishing the connection is up to the individual, Dr. Klinghardt makes sure that they have an important piece of information. "They need to know that from a neuropeptide perspective, every time you take drugs, it becomes more difficult for you to reach naturally that state of true and honest connection to God. You can't commune with God on drugs. You can get close to Him, but you'll never get there. Close to Him is like close to being pregnant or close to having an orgasm—it's not the real thing. So when addicts understand that the only way they can get there is sober and clean and not on drugs, and that every time they do something or take something, it pollutes the neuropeptides and the receptors more, and it gets more and more difficult to get there on their own, sometimes that cognitive information can help them commit to cleaning up."

Removing interference at the fifth level requires self-healing. Direct contact with nature is one way to reforge the connection with the Divine. "True prayer and true meditation work on this level as ways of getting there, but it's a level where there is no possibility of interaction between the healer and the patient," states Dr. Klinghardt. "I always say, if anybody tries to be helpful on this level, run as fast as you can." He notes that gurus and other spiritual teachers belong on the fourth level and have a valuable place there but have no business on the fifth level. If they trespass into that level, they are

Natural Medicine and the Five Levels of Healing

The chart below shows on what level the natural medicine therapeutic modalities in this book function.

Therapy	Level	Chapter
Amino Acid/ Neurotransmitter Restoration	Physical Body	3: The Biochemistry of Addiction
Applied Psychoneurobiology	Physical Body Electromagnetic Body Mental Body	7: The Five Levels of Healing
Family Systems Therapy	Intuitive Body	7: The Five Levels of Healing
Flower Essence Therapy	Mental Body	6: Energy Medicine II
NAET (allergy elimination)	Electromagnetic Body	4: Allergies and Addiction
Psychic Healing	Intuitive Body	9: Psychic Healing
Seemorg Matrix Work	Electromagnetic Body Mental Body	8: Energy, Trauma, and Spirit
Thought Field Therapy	Electromagnetic Body Mental Body	7: The Five Levels of Healing 8: Energy, Trauma, and Spirit
Traditional Chinese Medicine	Physical Body Electromagnetic Body	5: Energy Medicine I

putting themselves where God should be, says Dr. Klinghardt. "It's very dangerous."

That said, a number of the therapies in this book clear the impediments to spiritual connection that exist on other levels, especially the Mental and Intuitive, thus opening the way for individuals to reestablish balance for themselves on the fifth level. Using Applied Psychoneurobiology or Family Systems Therapy to discover and heal the source of disconnection from trust in God, which may be a psychological trauma (third-level factor) or a transgenerational legacy (fourth-level factor), is an example of this.

Operating Principles of the Five Healing Levels

The levels affect each other differently, depending on whether the influence is traveling upward or downward through them. Both trauma and successful therapeutic intervention at the higher levels have a rapid and deeply penetrating effect on the lower levels, says Dr. Klinghardt. This means that both the cause and the cure at the upper levels spread downward quickly. For example, if a systemic family issue is strongly present at the fourth (Intuitive) level, it will have profound effects on the first three levels. Similarly, resolving that issue can produce rapid changes in the Physical, Electromagnetic, and Mental Bodies. The lower levels may correct on their own, without further remediation.

At the same time, trauma or therapeutic intervention at the lower levels has a very slow and little penetrating effect upwards. When you get a physical injury (the first level), for instance, it will gradually change your electromagnetic field (the second level), altering the energy flow in your body. It's a slow process, however. The same is true for healing. "If you want to heal an injury on the second level— let's say you have a chakra that's blocked—you can do that by giving herbs and vitamins (biochemical interventions), but it will take years," says Dr. Klinghardt. But if you do an intervention on the third or fourth level, it can correct the blocked chakra on the second level immediately, within seconds or minutes, he notes.

The following case history illustrates the relationship between addiction and the levels of healing, and how the therapies Dr. Klinghardt uses can remove these interferences and bring addiction to a natural end.

Marcus: Smoking in Solidarity

Marcus, who was German, had already been smoking for years by the time he was 17, at which point his parents brought him to Dr. Klinghardt with the hopes that his methods would bring an end to the habit. "Being New Age people, it was the greatest embarrassment to them that a son was smoking," he recalls.

Marcus's history revealed nothing remarkable in relation to his smoking addiction, aside from the fact that he had mercury amalgam fillings, which might have been contributing to his addictive cravings. Muscle testing revealed the usual high levels of mercury in the brain, so Dr. Klinghardt put Marcus through his standard detoxification protocol, which uses DMPS, cilantro, chlorella, B vitamins, and vitamin C. Though he has found that fourth-level issues are usually the interference behind addiction, he has also discovered that until you get the mercury out, Family Systems Therapy or other methods won't be able to clear the fourth-level interference. The mercury creates a kind of wall that prevents the other therapies from working, Dr. Klinghardt explains. With the heavy metals removed, other interventions can be completed quickly and effectively.

Among the B vitamins Dr. Klinghardt gave Marcus was a high dose of niacin (vitamin B_3), 1000 mg three times a day. The reason for this vitamin in particular is that cigarette tobacco is a good source of niacin. This is borne out by the early Native American practice of sprinkling the leaves of the tobacco plant over their food, he explains, because their staples of beans, squash, and corn lacked niacin. "Some people actually crave smoking because they need the niacin. When you withdraw somebody from smoking, you have to know that you are also taking away B vitamins from them." For this reason, niacin needs to be an integral part of any detoxification program for smokers. As discussed in chapter 4, an allergy to B vitamins may prevent the absorption of these nutrients and produce a craving for them.

Marcus also had Thought Field Therapy treatments for the psychological aspect of his addiction. For this, Dr. Klinghardt tested his meridians while Marcus imagined how it felt to smoke, how bad he felt when he couldn't smoke, and how much he craved it. Any meridians that tested weak during this process were then treated with the tapping sequences of TFT (see "About the Therapies and Techniques").

At Marcus's five-month follow-up visit, he was completely off cigarettes and had been for some time, but he was depressed. At that point, Dr. Klinghardt introduced some APN work, which was soon focused on Marcus's grandfather, who had died in the Holocaust. A Protestant priest who resisted Nazi rule, he was shot in one of the concentration camps.

Marcus belonged to that German generation who identified with their grandparents and smoked in unconscious solidarity with their stand against Hitler, while that identification skipped their parents' generation (see sidebar). Note that Marcus's parents did not smoke and were opposed to it.

When through the APN session Marcus became aware of his identification with his grandfather, he broke down crying. He recognized how much he admired his grandfather, whom he had never had the chance to know, and how he had always revolted against any sort of authority. Smoking was part of that revolt. He saw that his parents were vegetarians, like Hitler, and did yoga and meditation, like Hitler, and were against smoking, as Hitler was. Marcus had thought that he was rebelling against his parents, but it was actually that he was identifying with and living the legacy of his grandfather. In his smoking, he was actually fighting the oppression of Hitler. "When he saw that, he cried for a long time," recalls Dr. Klinghardt.

According to the tenets of Family Systems Therapy, to remove the fourth-level interference that was causing his depression, Marcus needed to consciously establish the link with his grandfather. His smoking had masked the depression of carrying that legacy without being aware of the link. Using Applied Psychoneurobiology, Dr. Klinghardt induced in Marcus the mild hypnotic state that would allow him to connect with his grandparent in the psychic world and acknowledge him as one of his heroes.

That one session was sufficient to dispel Marcus's depression and end his smoking. That was ten years ago. Marcus is an attorney now and remains a nonsmoker.

About the Therapies and Techniques

Applied Psychoneurobiology (APN): This therapeutic technique was developed by Dr. Klinghardt. Employing his muscle testing method (see ART below) as a guide, APN uses stress signals in the autonomic nervous system to communicate with a patient's unconscious mind. "You can establish a code with the unconscious mind for yes and no in answer to questions," he explains. "The code is the strength or the weakness of a test muscle." APN can lead the way to the beliefs that underlie disorders such as addiction and exchange those beliefs with ones that promote balance in the Mental Body. This can produce dramatic shifts in the health and well-being of the person, notes Dr. Klinghardt.

Autonomic Response Testing (ART): ART, also called neural kinesiology, is a system of testing developed by Dr. Klinghardt. It employs a variety of methods, including muscle response testing (similar to that used in NAET, which is discussed in chapter 4) and arm length testing, to measure changes in the autonomic nervous system. (The autonomic nervous system controls the automatic processes of the body such as respiration, heart rate, digestion, and response to stress.) ART is used to identify distress in the body and determine optimum treatment. In general, a strong arm (or finger, depending on the kind of muscle testing) or an even arm length (in arm length testing) indicates that the system is not in distress. A weak muscle or uneven arm length indicates the presence of a factor that is causing stress to the client's organism.

Chelation: This is a therapy that removes heavy metals from the body, among other therapeutic functions. DMPS (2,3-dimercapto-propane-1-sulfonate) is a substance used as a chelating agent, which means that it binds with heavy metals, notably mercury, and is then excreted from the body. DMPS can be administered orally, intravenously, or intramuscularly. Other chelation agents are cilantro, chlorella, alpha lipoic acid, and glutathione.

NAET (Nambudripad's Allergy Elimination Techniques): NAET, developed by Devi S. Nambudripad, M.D., D.C., L.Ac., Ph.D., is a noninvasive and painless method for both identifying and eliminating allergies. It uses kinesiology's muscle response testing to identify allergies. Chiropractic and acupuncture techniques are then implemented to remove the energy blockages in the body that underlie allergies, and to reprogram the brain and nervous system not to respond allergically to previously problem substances. See chapter 4 for a full discussion of NAET.

Thought Field Therapy (TFT): Psychotherapist Roger J. Callahan,

Ph.D., developed TFT in response to his frustration at the failure of psychotherapy to help certain clients. It combines principles of acupuncture and psychology to heal the Mental Body. It actually operates on the boundary between the second and third levels, the Electromagnetic and the Mental Bodies, says Dr. Klinghardt. "The thought field is like a net that's attached on the outside of the electromagnetic field. Through early childhood trauma, the net is torn off the electric field."

TFT restores the attachment points between the electromagnetic and mental fields and restores the proper energy flow in the body's meridians. It accomplishes this through tapping gently with the fingertips on certain points on the skin. The particular series of tapping points is known as an algorithm. These are acupuncture points that also correspond to the attachment sites, which are slightly out from the body. The tapping functions similarly to the needles in acupuncture, which remove energy blockages and restore the flow of energy along the meridians. See chapter 8 for more about TFT.

For more information about the therapies or to locate a practitioner near you, see the following:

- APN, ART, and Neural Therapy: Dr. Klinghardt (see appendix); websites: www.neuraltherapy.com and www.pnf.org/neural_kinesiology.html.
- Chelation: The American College for Advancement in Medicine (ACAM), 23121 Verdugo Drive, Suite 204, Laguna Hills, CA 92653; fax: 949-455-9679; website: www.acam.org.
- NAET: Devi S. Nambudripad, M.D., D.C., L.Ac., Ph.D., Pain Clinic, 6714 Beach Boulevard, Buena Park, CA 90621; tel: 714-523-8900; website: www.naet.com; also see her book *Say Good-Bye to Illness* (Buena Park, CA: Delta Publishing, 1999).
- TFT: *Tapping the Healer Within*, by Roger J. Callahan, Ph.D. (Chicago: Contemporary Books, 2001); for a practitioner, contact the Callahan Techniques office, 78-816 Via Carmel, La Quinta, CA 92253; tel: 760-360-7832; website: www.tftrx.com (professional site), www.selfhelpuniv.com (self-help site).

8 Energy, Trauma, and Spirit: Thought Field Therapy and Seemorg Matrix Work

While we have seen in this book that many factors that contribute to addiction are not addressed by psychotherapy, we have also seen that psychospiritual issues and the energy disturbances they create can play a role and may need to be attended to for long-lasting recovery. This chapter explores two psychotherapeutic techniques: Thought Field Therapy (TFT) and Seemorg Matrix Work.

Rather than focusing on verbal processing of psychospiritual issues, these methods are energy-based psychotherapies. Their operating premise is that disturbances in an individual's energy field underlie addiction, anxiety and depression (again, both of which are frequently present in addiction), and other symptoms and conditions. Such disturbances can be caused by "energy toxins" or psychospiritual trauma. By clearing the energy field, resolution of the condition can be achieved. These methods are much faster than standard psychotherapy and address the underlying energy problems, which the latter does not. Hundreds of therapists have been trained in both of these techniques as word of their effectiveness has spread.

More about Thought Field Therapy

As discussed in the previous chapter, Thought Field Therapy works in the body's Thought Field (the Mental Body in Dr.

Klinghardt's model). Blocked or disturbed energy flow in this field is corrected through tapping on certain acupuncture points on the body while the client thinks of the situations, events, or objects that trigger anxiety or other distress; or in the case of addiction, the client thinks about the addictive cravings or the feeling when indulging in the addictive substance or activity. People who suffer from addictions can learn to self-administer TFT and use it whenever they feel cravings or the anxiety underlying their addictive urges.

Clinical psychologist Roger J. Callahan, Ph.D., the founder of TFT and the author of a number of books including *The Anxiety-Addiction Connection: Eliminate Your Addictive Urges with Thought Field Therapy,* maintains that addiction is actually an attempt to tranquilize anxiety. "All addiction problems are a result of the anxiety-masking effect of certain drugs . . . or the anxiety-masking effect of certain activities. . . . [230] In the category of drugs, he includes caffeine, tobacco, chocolate, and food in general, as well as legal and illegal drugs. Among many activities, he cites nail biting, hair pulling, and the obsessive rituals of severe anxiety disorders (such as obsessive-compulsive disorder), which have an addictive component.

The operative word here is "masking" because the addictive substances and activities do not resolve the anxiety, says Dr. Callahan, but rather "sweep the anxiety under the rug where it festers and grows worse, setting the stage for the need for more and more drugs to disguise the ever increasing anxiety."

The operative word here is "masking," because the addictive substances and activities do not resolve the anxiety, says Dr. Callahan, but rather "sweep the anxiety under the rug where it festers and grows worse, setting the stage for the need for more and more drugs to disguise the ever increasing anxiety."[231]

Dr. Callahan contends that cravings and withdrawal symptoms are an outgrowth of the anxiety, which is supported by the fact that supposedly physiologically addictive drugs such as heroin have proven to be nonaddictive and do not produce withdrawal symptoms after a period of use to relieve physical pain, for example.[232] In these cases, anxiety was not the motivating factor in the drug use. Dr. Callahan's theory is further supported by the fact that TFT, which is well known for its efficacy in eliminating anxiety and panic attacks, effectively reduces or ends cravings and withdrawal symptoms.

By Dr. Callahan's model, the alarming rise in both anxiety disorders and addiction in the past few decades is not a parallel occurrence but an interrelated phenomenon. In his view, the failure to address the underlying anxiety is the reason for the abysmal success rate of most addiction treatment programs.[233]

For more about anxiety, see my book *The Natural Medicine Guide to Anxiety* (Hampton Roads, 2003).

The operating principle of TFT is that anxiety, and thus addiction, is a manifestation of an energy perturbation in the acupuncture meridian system (see chapters 5 and 7). In other words, some disturbance has thrown your energy system out of balance. Dr. Callahan was a pioneer in cognitive therapy, a form of "talk" therapy that focuses on retraining the mind out of old patterns in order to produce emotional and behavioral changes. His research and clinical experience over time led him to rethink his approach, and the result was TFT.

"Many experts in the mental health field today believe that chemistry or cognitions are the fundamental cause of disturbed emotions," states Dr. Callahan. "The basic premise of Thought Field Therapy, however, is that the perturbation(s) in the thought field precedes and generates these chemical and cognitive facts."[234] The response of patients to TFT supports the energy model. Dr. Callahan claims a 75- to 80-percent success rate, meaning that "75 to 80 percent of people can expect to have their negative emotions [such as anxiety] completely resolved."[235] For the elimination of addictive cravings alone, the rate is even higher. Dr. Callahan places TFT's success rate in this area at about 90 percent.[236]

According to the TFT model, the perturbations, or disturbances, in the energy field often result from energy toxins, or allergies, sensitivities, or intolerances, as they are variously termed. The phrase "energy toxin" reflects how the offending substance can throw the energy system out of balance. Heavy metal and chemical toxicities fall into the category of energy toxins as well.

Both the TFT and Seemorg Matrix Work models recognize that psychological trauma can also create energy perturbations. "Traumatic experiences in childhood, in the womb, even in past lives or in your heritage, can be the source of aberrations in a person's energy field," explains Tony Roffers, Ph.D., of Oakland, California, who is versed in both methods. A psychotherapist for over 30 years, he has expertise in a range of psychotherapeutic modalities. In recent years, he began using Thought Field Therapy and Seemorg Matrix Work and was so impressed by the results that they are now the centerpieces of his practice.

In TFT, it is not necessary to determine the cause of the energy aberration or gain insight into your anxiety, as is the traditional approach in psychotherapy, Dr. Roffers explains. "The only insight you need is that there was something messed up in your meridians that has now been fixed, and you now know how to fix it on your own if you need to."

This runs counter to the approach of the majority of traditional psychotherapists, he observes, which is why many regard TFT as not a true therapy because it doesn't lead to understanding or insight that could have application to other aspects of the client's life. "The notion that insight is a necessary prerequisite for behavioral change is a very strong notion in Western psychology. I personally have gone through quite a transformation about that, in the sense that I think insight is often an *important* prerequisite, and does aid in the generalization of therapeutic work to other arenas of the client's life, but I no longer see it as a *necessary* prerequisite," states Dr. Roffers.

"Insight assumes that the mind, one's awareness, can influence one's behavior and can lead you to the heart of the matter," but according to Thought Field Therapy, "a perturbation in the thought field is at the heart of the matter. This perturbation serves as a trigger for all kinds of aberrations that are on neurological, hormonal, chemical, and cognitive levels." In other words, an energy disturbance can produce all kinds of physical and mental symptoms, and if you resolve the issue in the energy field, the symptoms go away. (Note

that this is the basis of traditional Chinese medicine as well;
see chapter 5.)

If TFT doesn't work, it is
typically because something you
are eating, breathing, or being
exposed to reinstates the energy
perturbation, or an early trauma
that has not been uncovered or
treated is keeping the energy
problem in place, explains Dr.
Roffers. In these cases, allergy
identification and elimination
techniques such as NAET (see
chapters 4 and 7) and psychotherapeutic methods such as
Seemorg Matrix Work (see the
next section in this chapter) may
be necessary to resolve the disturbance.

In Their Own Words

*"[Meth] is like a companion
telling you that you're good
enough, handsome enough,
and smart enough, banishing all
the little insecurities to your subconscious, liberating you from
self doubts yet making you feel
completely alive. . . . When I
stopped smoking for a few days
just to see if I could, a profound
depression would overcome me.
Nothing seemed worthwhile."*
—magazine writer
Karl Taro Greenfeld[238]

There is another phenomenon which is particularly operational
in addiction. While TFT works well to eliminate cravings and it is
easy to teach people how to do it themselves, Dr. Callahan has found
that many people won't do it when they are feeling addictive urges.
Why not? "Because the addiction process creates a self-sabotaging
state in the addict that I call psychological reversal," states Dr.
Callahan. "This state makes it especially difficult to overcome the
addiction because it drives the addict to engage in self-defeating and
self-sabotaging activities and to become his own worst enemy."[237]

According to the TFT model, psychological reversal blocks treatment and prevents recovery from addiction. Psychological reversal
can happen in any disorder, but it is far more prevalent among people with addictions. In fact, it is nearly universal in this group. Dr.
Callahan developed a tapping procedure to correct psychological
reversal, and it is usually necessary for people with addictions to perform this on themselves frequently.

Dr. Roffers sums up psychological reversal in this way: "Whatever
you desire the most or whatever you want to do, particularly if it's in a

constructive, positive direction, unconsciously or consciously you find yourself doing the exact opposite or in some way undermining it."

His clinical experience confirms Dr. Callahan's observations regarding the prevalence of this problem in addiction. "People who have addictions are full of recurring reversals, to the point where you have to have them clear the reversals throughout the day. They have to be constantly aligning themselves or they won't even use the addiction algorithm [tapping sequence] to reduce their addictive craving because they're reversed and they just say, 'To hell with it.'" The tapping sequence corrects the psychological reversal, realigning the person in an energetic sense, by restoring balance to his or her energy field.

Dr. Roffers postulates that the reason why reversal is such a problem in addiction is that multiple energy toxins (allergens and chemical toxicities) are present and these create nearly constant energy perturbations. Clearing energy toxins is an integral part of his work. For this, he has found Seemorg Matrix Work most effective. It also works to clear the psychological issues and core beliefs that contribute to psychological reversal, anxiety, and addiction in general.

 For help locating a TFT practitioner, contact the Callahan Techniques office, 78-816 Via Carmel, La Quinta, CA 92253; tel: 760-360-7832; website: www.tftrx.com (professional site), www.selfhelpuniv.com (self-help site). For information about Seemorg Matrix Work, contact Asha Nahoma Clinton, L.C.S.W., Ph.D., Energy Revolution, Inc., 885 East Road, Richmond, MA 01254; tel: 413-698-2744; e-mail: energyrev@ seemorgmatrix.org; website: www.seemorgmatrix.org. The website has a directory of practitioners.

What Is Seemorg Matrix Work?

Psychotherapist Asha Nahoma Clinton, L.C.S.W., Ph.D., developed Seemorg Matrix Work in the mid-1990s as a result of her dissatisfaction with the results produced by psychodynamic psychotherapy, which she had been practicing for 20 years. Matrix Work is "the first transpersonal, body-centered energy psychother-

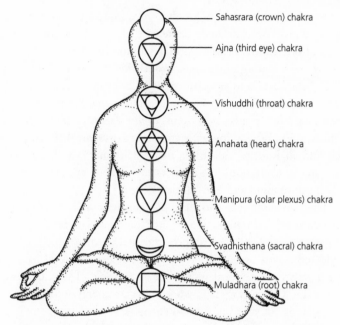

- Sahasrara (crown) chakra
- Ajna (third eye) chakra
- Vishuddhi (throat) chakra
- Anahata (heart) chakra
- Manipura (solar plexus) chakra
- Svadhisthana (sacral) chakra
- Muladhara (root) chakra

The Seven Major Chakras or Body Energy Vortexes

apy," to quote Dr. Clinton. "It treats trauma and its many psychological, physical, intellectual, and spiritual aftereffects with the movement of energy through the major energy centers."[239]

The transpersonal psychotherapy aspect of Seemorg Matrix Work is found in its focus on "removing the blocks that impede spiritual development" and "a spiritual technology to nurture and enhance that development."[240] Its name reflects this orientation; Seemorg, a fabulous bird featured in ancient Middle Eastern and Indian tales, is a symbol of the Divine.[241]

The major energy centers to which Dr. Clinton refers are the chakras, the series of seven energy vortexes positioned along the midline of the body from the base of the spine to the crown of the head, as discussed previously in the book. As noted in chapter 7, when chakras are blocked, the free flow of energy in the body's field is impeded. Matrix Work uses the chakra system, progressing from top to bottom, to move negative energy out of the body. It then proceeds through the chakras from bottom to top, bringing positive energy into the body. This is the body-centered energy aspect of the therapy.

Dr. Roffers works closely with Dr. Clinton and, next to her, is the most versed Seemorg practitioner worldwide. He explains the relevance of the chakras to psychotherapy: "The chakras are like switchboards for the meridian system, central energy centers for this electromagnetic circulatory system in the body. Seemorg Matrix Work is a way of working with your energy system that can put it back into alignment." According to Dr. Clinton's model, trauma is the source of aberrations in a person's energy field, and those aberrations produce mind and body disorders.

There are essentially two kinds of traumas, says Dr. Roffers. One is the crisis type of trauma, as in your father beat you or you fell off the garage roof. The other is developmental trauma, which is more subtle and occurs over a period of time. The experience of having a distant father or a critical mother is an example of developmental trauma. Dr. Clinton's therapy works with the energy system to clear those traumas in your body on an energetic level. With the traumas cleared and the energy balance restored, the disorders that stemmed from the energy aberration can self-correct.

The Matrix approach works in "a much more holistic, integrated way than the traditional talking therapy," states Dr. Roffers. It also significantly reduces the healing time, although it is still not a quick fix. "The metaphor I use is if you're going to remodel your kitchen and someone starts going into the walls and finds out where a leak is, pretty soon the whole kitchen may be torn apart." It can be like that when the "kitchen" is the patient's psyche.

As noted above, the therapy can also be used to clear energy toxins (allergies), which is an important intervention in cases of addiction. According to the Seemorg Matrix model, trauma is at the root of many allergies; the hypothesis is that the substance was in the person's energy field when the trauma occurred, and so the person developed "disharmony" with that substance. The disharmony can be reversed by reintroducing the substance into the person's field and using Matrix Work to move through all the chakras, removing the aftereffects of trauma and realigning the energy.

Dr. Roffers notes that regardless of how the allergy began,

whether the hypothesis holds true or not, "aligning the meridians and the chakras in this way strengthens the person's system, aligns them, or puts them more in harmony with whatever the substance is." He adds, "I'm getting better results clearing energy toxins using Matrix Work, and specifically the clearing of traumas, than with any of the other methods I've used." Dr. Roffers is trained in several other energy-based allergy elimination techniques.

"Modern-Day Exorcism"

Dr. Roffers calls Matrix Work "modern-day exorcism." This is a reference to the legitimate and effective energy work that exorcism, as performed by skilled shamans of old, entailed. Matrix Work removes the energy influences to which we are subject today.

The work begins with the practitioner taking a thorough history, including what is known as a "trauma history." For the latter, clients list whatever traumas, of both the crisis and developmental types, they can remember.

To monitor the status of energy in the body throughout the work that follows, the therapist uses kinesiological muscle testing. For this, you hold one arm straight out in front of you and attempt to keep it there while the practitioner pushes down slightly on your wrist. Normally, you can easily hold your arm in place, but when there is an energy disturbance in your meridian system, the muscle response is weakened. While you are being tested, the practitioner has you think of the trauma or asks you to make specific statements.

First, however, the practitioner tests you to make sure that you are not "neurologically disorganized." Other terms or phrases for this condition are "switched," being in "massive reversal," or having your "polarization off," states Dr. Roffers. Regardless of the term, the upshot is that if you are in this state, muscle testing will not be reliable.

To check for neurological disorganization, you place either hand on top of your head with the palm down, then extend your other arm out in front of you for the practitioner to test as in the standard muscle testing, Dr. Roffers explains. If the arm tests strong, the body is in alignment. When you turn the palm of the hand on your head up instead of down, the extended arm should test weak, because that position takes the body out of alignment. Any other combination (such as when the palm is down, the arm is weak; or when the palm is up, the arm is strong) is a reversal, a sign of neurological disorganization. The practitioner must then use a technique to realign the person so muscle testing will be accurate.

The next step in the Matrix process is the Covenant. The therapist starts by asking the client to say, "I give permission for my being to be healed." If the arm response on that is weak, it means the person is not giving permission. "You have to clear that, or they're not ready to be treated," Dr. Roffers states. "By clearing any negative beliefs that get in the way of treating traumas, the Covenant is a way of assuring that the person is going to be open to the treatment and, once you treat traumas, that those treatments will hold."

To clear the negative belief, you hold a hand over each chakra in turn, going from top to bottom, repeating the belief at each chakra. The therapist then conducts the muscle testing again to make sure that the negative statement has cleared from the body. A positive belief about the treatment (for example, "I can be healed") is then instilled in the same way, but by going up the chakras, from bottom to top.

While one hand moves from chakra to chakra, the other maintains a position over the primary chakra for that particular person, which is determined via muscle testing. The primary chakra is called the stationary point. Dr. Roffers observes that for traumas many people need to hold the heart chakra, but it can be the solar plexus or another chakra. For negative beliefs, the primary chakra is usually the "third-eye" point (sixth chakra) on the forehead.

The client keeps one hand on the primary chakra throughout the process. "The two hands create an electromagnetic loop," he explains. "My hypothesis is that by closing that electromagnetic loop, you're realigning something in the body that's been misaligned and, as you clear that loop, something shifts. Then when you go to the next level, something else shifts." You will find that some chakras don't have any misalignment in them, he adds.

After the Covenant is completed, the therapist moves to clearing traumas, first identifying the primary chakra (stationary point) and a phrase that describes the trauma (for example, "My father abandoned me"). The client then moves down through the chakras, repeating the phrase at each.

There is no rigid order in proceeding with Seemorg Matrix Work because it is tailored to the client, notes Dr. Roffers, but generally the focus at this point turns to the originating traumas. These are the traumas that occurred very early in life. To clarify the nature of trauma, Dr. Clinton offers the following definition:

> A trauma is any occurrence which, when we think of it or it is triggered by some present event, evokes difficult emotions and/or physical symptoms, gives rise to negative beliefs, desire, fantasies, compulsions, obsessions, addictions or dissociation, blocks the development of positive qualities and spiritual connection, and fractures human wholeness.[242]

After working with the originating traumas, the focus shifts to the initiatory traumas, usually the events that brought the person into therapy. "These are the much more recent traumas," explains Dr. Roffers, "which are a retraumatization of the originating traumas."

Next is to clear the connections between the originating and initiatory traumas, and then the traumatic patterns. The latter are like a web of traumas that gets woven around an originating trauma; you could also call this web a syndrome of traumas. For example, "if you had a very cold and distant father, you selectively attend to men who are that way, and you begin to attract men who are cold and distant, as a misguided attempt to heal," says Dr. Roffers. The belief, "All men are cold and distant," is formed secondarily as a result of the originating and subsequent traumas.

The next step is to clear the negative or dysfunctional beliefs that have accrued as a result of traumas and instill the more positive or functional beliefs using the Core Belief Matrix. "A matrix is a cluster of interrelated core beliefs around a certain trauma," explains Dr. Roffers. A Core Belief Matrix is a series of statements, stated first in the negative and then in the positive, that reflect core beliefs. An example of a negative statement in a Matrix is "I can be used," while the corresponding positive statement is "I will no longer permit being used."

The client says each negative statement in turn, with the therapist conducting muscle testing. When a person says, "I can be used," and the arm response is strong, it means the person believes that statement.

Before proceeding to the next statement, "you have to take that dysfunctional belief out," says Dr. Roffers. The client goes down the chakras, saying the negative core belief. Then the corresponding positive core belief—"I will no longer permit being used"—is instilled by going up the chakras, repeating the positive statement at each chakra with one hand placed on the third-eye chakra (between the eyes) as the stationary point.

By clearing the traumas, traumatic patterns, and negative core beliefs and realigning the attendant energy imbalance, a condition such as anxiety, along with the addictions used to mask it, can be resolved. As with other energy-based modalities, correcting the energy flow often results in self-correction of factors that present in anxiety and addiction and may seem to be causal factors, such as neurotransmitter imbalances.

As stated previously, another corollary of Seemorg Matrix Work is that it tends to open people up to spiritual possibilities. "To me, it's a major answer to how psychological work integrates with spiritual development," says Dr. Roffers. "If you have trauma, it separates you from God. It separates you from yourself. It separates you from others. It separates you from the Earth, the universe."

Clearing traumas and the self-sabotaging negative beliefs that cluster around them enables you "to become more whole within yourself, and you're much more open and permeable and interested in working on that spiritual level." Given that the source of addiction is often an interference on the spiritual level, this development can be an important component in treatment.

Having worked extensively with the Matrix method, Dr. Roffers now believes that this clearing can be done for most people and for most types of trauma. The following case histories from Dr. Roffers' files demonstrate how Thought Field Therapy and Matrix Work can be used in combination to resolve addiction.

Mike: Smoking and Sex Addiction

Mike came to Dr. Roffers when he was in his early forties. He had been smoking since his early twenties. He had tried everything to stop smoking and had managed to for short periods over the years, but had never been able to maintain it. It wasn't just the smoking that had prompted him to seek help, however. Mike was living two lives, one of them in secret. On the surface, he was a seeming happily married man who was embarking on a new and more meaningful career track as a chiropractor. Unbeknownst to anyone in that life, he had a whole other world. In thrall to a sadomasochistic sex addiction, he regularly visited dominatrices.

He was ashamed of what he was doing and had tried to stop, but could not. Dr. Roffers was the first person that Mike had told about this. He was in the midst of training to be a chiropractor and felt that he could not in good conscience work as a healthcare practitioner unless he overcame his addictions.

When Dr. Roffers first started working with Mike, it was before he had discovered Matrix Work. He used Rational Emotive Behavior Therapy (which focuses on replacing thoughts, feelings, and actions that do not serve the best interests of the individual with ones that do; cognitive therapy and cognitive-behavioral therapy grew out of this method[243]) to uncover the inner beliefs that might be informing his addictions. This helped to some degree but didn't produce any lasting change.

At that point, Dr. Roffers had started using Thought Field Therapy, and he taught Mike the tapping sequences that he could do on himself when he felt the addictive urges, both for cigarettes and the sadomasochistic sex. When Mike did the tapping, it worked, but "he was the classic addiction person," recalls Dr. Roffers. "He either would forget to do the tapping that would reduce the craving, or would say, 'Screw it. If I do that, I might not have a smoke or go to whoever I want to do my S&M stuff with.'"

As with most people with addictions, he was constantly in this state of psychological reversal, sabotaging his best intentions and desires. When Dr. Roffers taught him the procedure to align himself and get rid of the reversal, things began to get better. Mike performed this procedure many times during the day, and so when the addictive cravings arose, he was willing to do the tapping. He became able to stop himself from going to the dominatrices, but he was still obsessing about it. "The compulsive behavior stopped," notes Dr. Roffers, "but the obsessive thoughts didn't."

He had significantly reduced his smoking by then but hadn't stopped completely and would smoke whenever he felt anxious. At that point, Dr. Roffers introduced Seemorg Matrix Work. As testing revealed that Mike had allergies to grains and dairy, he integrated the energy toxin work with clearing the traumas.

"The originating traumas, the earliest ones we could find, were with both mother and father. His was a very complicated case, but the highlights of it were that he had an extremely abusive mother, physically as well as verbally, and an alcoholic father who was a reasonably okay guy when he wasn't on alcohol, but when he was drinking, became very irresponsible, judgmental, and critical."

Dr. Roffers summarizes what the therapies accomplished in Mike's case: "The TFT got the addictive behavior—the sex addiction—under control. The matrix work cleared the underlying parts of the iceberg that needed to be cleared to resolve his masochism."

The core beliefs connected to Mike's early trauma were that he was "a piece of shit." His severe self-judgment was, "I'm no good. I never will be any good. I'm bad. I deserve to be punished." He had internalized the view his parents had projected onto him. Mike already knew this from the earlier therapy, but it had not made a difference to know it. "Only when we were able to clear the traumas around that and some of those beliefs" did significant change occur, notes Dr. Roffers.

Mike had about four months of Matrix Work to clear his complicated web of traumas. During that time, he stopped smoking and stopped his sexual addiction patterns.

Dr. Roffers summarizes what the therapies accomplished in his case: "The TFT got the addictive behavior—the sex addiction—under control. The matrix work cleared the underlying parts of the iceberg that needed to be cleared to resolve his masochism."

Dr. Roffers ran a check with Mike recently. He asked, "Have you gone back to any of these women?"

Mike answered that it had been two years since he visited a dominatrix.

"What about the obsessive thinking?" asked Dr. Roffers.

"Every once in a while," said Mike, adding that the last time had been when his younger brother was told that he had cancer of the liver and might not last the year. It shook his whole sense of solidity in the world. He took a walk to calm down and "had some of those thoughts again," referring to thinking about sadomasochistic sex. But it was very manageable, nonobsessive, and "not that interesting." He didn't even need to do the tapping. He just observed that that was what was happening and then started worrying about his brother.

In Mike's case, his addictions were an attempt to self-medicate generalized anxiety (anxiety for no apparent reason) and social phobia that manifested in high levels of anxiety whenever he went to a social gathering or had to present to his classmates in chiropractic school. "Once the traumas underlying his addictions were clear, he no longer needed to self-medicate," explains Dr. Roffers.

Dirk: Grain Allergies, Trauma, and Alcoholism

Dirk had begun drinking heavily in his teens, and alcohol had been a part of his life ever since. While he was in his twenties, he still considered his drinking merely youthful excess, but now in his thirties he had recently faced the fact that he was a full-blown alcoholic. Having heard of Dr. Roffer's work in the area of addictions, he came to him for help. He had just stopped drinking but was having an extremely hard time staying away from alcohol.

In Dirk's case, his addiction stemmed from "trauma with his father in combination with a lot of grain allergies," says Dr. Roffers. In his clinical experience, the latter is typical of alcoholism. "Alcoholism, for me, is just a carbohydrate addiction," he states. "People substitute cola or coffee or sweets for the alcohol, but it doesn't change their basic metabolic structure. You've got to get them off all that sort of stuff, and you need amino acids to help them to do that." The reason for avoiding these foods and beverages is that they cause low blood sugar, which in turn produces more cravings.

 For more about amino acids, see chapter 3.

Dr. Roffers gave Dirk the amino acid L-glutamine to reduce his carbohydrate cravings and therefore his desire for a drink, and 5-HTP (5-hydroxy tryptophan) to promote the production of serotonin. He also took him off all grains, due to his allergies. As further assistance in avoiding alcohol, he did Thought Field Therapy with him and taught him the tapping sequences to reduce cravings and to clear the psychological reversal that interferes with treatment and the intention to stop drinking.

With this basic program in place, Dr. Roffers proceeded to Matrix Work to clear the energy toxins (allergens) and the trauma underlying Dirk's alcoholism. One of the goals in eliminating the allergies was so Dirk could eat a more varied diet and better maintain his blood glucose level.

Dirk's early trauma was developmental in nature, meaning that it occurred over time, rather than in specific traumatic incidents. His parents had divorced when he was young, and his father had always had unrealistic needs when it came to his son. Dirk never felt like he could meet those needs, "and rightfully so, because they were unrealistic," comments Dr. Roffers. The core belief connected with this developmental trauma was "I'll never be good enough." This could be seen as the source of the anxiety that the alcohol served to mask.

In his life, Dirk perpetuated that belief by setting himself up with friends and girlfriends who would continually have unrealistic expectations of him. Matrix Work cleared the original negative belief and instilled a positive one in its place: "My father had unrealistic expectations of me." With that new belief instilled, Dirk would stop perpetuating the old pattern.

"That's what's changing now," notes Dr. Roffers. "He's able to discern better when people have unrealistic expectations of him. He doesn't walk into a relationship thinking, 'I'll never be good enough.'"

To clear all the associated traumas and core beliefs took about six months of Matrix Work. Dirk was able to stay off alcohol during that time, and it has now been a year and a half since he's had a drink.

9 Psychic Healing

While psychic healing may seem to be in an entirely different category from the other therapies covered in this book, it is actually another form of energy medicine that addresses disturbances in an individual's electromagnetic or energy field and, in so doing, brings body, mind, and spirit back into alignment. While each energy-based therapy, from acupuncture to Seemorg Matrix Work, has its own method for dealing with energy disturbances, the goal is the same: the clearing of negative influences and blockages and the restoration of balance, wholeness, and connectedness.

The negative influences and blockages addressed by psychic healing are found in the energy field that surrounds the body, which is also called the aura. While, unlike psychics, laypeople cannot typically see their aura, they receive evidence of its existence all the time. Have you ever "felt your skin crawl" when you met someone new? Have you ever suddenly and for no apparent reason felt drained or depressed when you walked into a room of people? These reactions are the result of discordant foreign energies entering your energy field, or aura, where they are not a good match with your energy and consequently produce a sense of unease or discomfort.

Unfortunately, energy influences are not just transitory. The energy field around your body is subtle and fragile and can actually be damaged, which renders it more permeable to foreign energies and more likely that they will remain. Among the events or practices that can damage or pollute the aura are emotional or physical trauma, psychic or verbal abuse, other people's negative or bad thoughts about you, and substance abuse. Obviously, the latter has particular relevance in the case of addiction.

Physicians and psychics alike have noted that the energy field can be poisoned or polluted by harmful energies that produce mental, emotional, and physical symptoms and, if allowed to remain, can lead to disease.[244]

Psychiatrist Shakuntala Modi, M.D., of Wheeling, West Virginia, has been researching energy field disturbances for over 15 years. She has identified a range of physical and psychological symptoms and conditions that result from such disturbances, from panic disorders and depression to headaches, weight gain, stammering, and even schizophrenia. Further, under clinical hypnotherapy (a form of therapy that involves inducing a hypnotic, or trancelike, state in the patient in order to access the unconscious mind), 77 out of 100 patients cited foreign "beings" in their aura as responsible for the symptoms or condition for which they were pursuing treatment. Dr. Modi's research revealed that these beings (foreign energies) are "the single leading cause of psychiatric problems."[245] Dr. Modi also found that after removing the foreign energies from the patient's energy field using hypnotherapy, the patient's symptoms "often cleared up immediately."[246]

The concept of energy disturbances in a person's energy field causing a variety of physical and psychological problems is gaining greater recognition and acceptance in the healing professions and among the public at large. A simple way to look at the issue of "energy pollution" is that, like the environment and your body, your energy field is subject to toxic buildup and requires cleansing to restore it to health. Just as we take measures to clean up our planet and engage in various body detoxification methods such as fasts or colonics, we need to take steps to clear the toxins from our auras. Psychic healing is a method for cleansing your energy field of the toxins that are interfering with your physical, emotional, and spiritual health.

What Is Psychic Healing?

Reverend Leon S. LeGant, a psychic healer based in San Francisco, California, concurs with Dr. Modi's research findings regarding the presence of foreign "beings." In the ten years that he has been working as a psychic healer, he has cleared hundreds of people of these disruptive influences in their energy fields. Among those who have sought his help have been substance abusers (of everything from alcohol to cocaine), though that problem was often not what brought them to LeGant. Through his work with them, he has learned that there tend to be certain types of "beings" that are present in people with addictions. Before we go into the details of his discoveries, let's look at what psychic healing is.

Simply put, a psychic is someone who is sensitive to nonphysical forces, explains LeGant. Psychic healing involves the removal of foreign energy (a nonphysical force) from your energy field. In addition to working with individual clients, LeGant is now devoting much of his time to training others in this type of healing. He is the director of the Psychic School, a nonprofit organization dedicated to the development of psychic abilities.

LeGant, who has been a clairvoyant all his life, believes that everyone is psychic to some degree. Their abilities vary depending on when they shut themselves down, which most people do between the ages of three and five in response to parental and societal invalidation of the spirit realm, he says.

LeGant defines clairvoyance as "the ability to see energy in the form of mental image pictures. Since everything in the universe is made of energy, you can see it clairvoyantly in the form of a symbol or image or a picture that would make sense to the person seeing the information or the image." He notes that, without the proper context for the visions, clairvoyance is easily labeled hallucination.

Childhood fears of the dark, of monsters in the closet, of things under the bed actually have foundation in reality, arising as they do from children's "clairvoyance sensing an energy in the room with them." Since it is frightening, they begin to turn off their clairvoyance, explains LeGant. The programming of the educational system and usually their parents as well support this suppression. "There's no validation for clairvoyance or being sensitive," he notes.

The imaginary friends of childhood also indicate children's connection to the spirit realm. These friends are their spirit guides. Again, messages from outside invalidate what children know to be true and teach them that "what they're sensing and seeing is not real, it's just an illusion or something they're making up." In most families, growing up requires that you stop having tea with your imaginary friends.

For some people, suppressing contact with the spirit realm is more difficult than for others. Psychics actually have "slightly different neurochemistry," LeGant explains. "Their pineal gland [located in the brain] is usually a little larger, and there may be a genetic component to it that affects their brain chemistry and allows them to process energy in the form of images and thoughts in their mind." In adolescence, the brain chemistry shifts, and the clairvoyance becomes highly active again. It takes that amount of time for the body to develop and be able to receive the information. Around the time that the neurochemistry changes is when psychics become hypersensitive. They can easily be overwhelmed by everything they are taking in and all that they are feeling as a result. "It's a lot to process," says LeGant, who speaks from personal experience.

A "grounded psychic" can balance between the physical and spiritual worlds and distinguish them from each other, but few psychics are assisted in accomplishing this until they are adults and are fortunate enough to find the help they need in handling their abilities. This has implications for addiction. Like those who suffer from depression, people with addictions (who frequently suffer from depression as well) share the psychic characteristic of hypersensitivity.

Addiction and Foreign Energies

Anyone with a mental disorder, and addiction is classified as such, is being influenced on some level through their spiritual sensitivity, says LeGant. Most people with addictions are highly sensitive. "They get overwhelmed with energy and other people's emotions, problems, and pain. They're very psychic, and they don't know how to handle it."

Pain is stuck energy, and when you absorb it, it weighs you down. "Someone who gets that overwhelmed and flooded with foreign energy leaves their body," LeGant notes. In psychotherapeutic terms, this is known as dissociation, mentally separating yourself from your body when the pain you feel is too great to stay present.

People often experience it as feeling "spaced out." In psychic terms, less of the person's awareness "leaves" the body than occurs during an out-of-body experience. The person may be slightly out of their body as long as the foreign energy or pain of trauma is present.

Regardless of the fact that the mind has checked out and is no longer aware of the foreign energy, the body continues to absorb others' pain (stuck energy), and its own energy flow becomes blocked. The person's own pain from past trauma adds to the mix, and for highly sensitive people who have no tools for dealing with all that is overwhelming them it is nearly unbearable.

One coping strategy people use is to self-medicate, turning to drugs and other substances in an attempt to numb out their sensitivity and stop the pain. While this may seem to work at first, it actually sets up a cycle of increasing pain, LeGant explains. "All that pain is still there, and the body is in a stuck space." Drug and other substance abuse knocks people out of their bodies, as described, leaving them more open to occupation by foreign energies,

Anyone with a mental disorder, and addiction is classified as such, is being influenced on some level through their spiritual sensitivity, says LeGant. Most people with addictions are highly sensitive. "They get overwhelmed with energy and other people's emotions, problems, and pain. They're very psychic, and they don't know how to handle it."

which in turn creates more internal pain. "When the drugs wear off, they start to feel the problems and the pain even more. They want to take more drugs to get back out of that again, and it starts this vicious cycle. The longer they stay addicted, the longer they use, the thicker the pain 'ridges' become, and the more difficult it is for them to clear that and get out of the cycle."

In addition, substance abuse actually damages the user's energy field. LeGant is able to identify what substance the person is using by the type of damage he sees in that individual's energy field. He typically doesn't know about the substance abuse, as noted above, but as he is psychically "reading" the person, he sees this damage, usually in the energy field of the brain, as that is where drugs and alcohol operate. "There's a different energy frequency with the different drugs," he notes.

With marijuana, there is a kind of "numbed-out" or "sticky" energy. With LSD, there is usually damage around the limbic system in the brain. "[The drug] ecstasy is really easy to spot. It puts holes in the brain," states LeGant, adding that these holes are apparent in CAT scans of the brains of people who have used a lot of ecstasy. Cocaine, crack, and speed are all in one category, and it's difficult to tell them apart. "I'll usually see a kind of 'wiring,' like silver webbing, in the brain," he observes, adding that it is almost as though these drugs are rewiring the brain. Alcohol, tranquilizers, and painkillers all produce a similar effect, "a numbed-out, whitish-blue energy all over the body."

The "Beings" in Your Energy Field

The foreign "beings" in the energy field of people who abuse drugs or alcohol feed off of those addictions. To understand how foreign "beings" or unfriendly spirits can occupy your energy field in the first place, it is necessary to consider life forms in the dimensions or realms beyond the third dimension in which we live.

"Fifth dimensional life forms are angels and the various beings of the angelic hierarchy. The fifth dimension is what most religions and forms of spirituality would consider heaven," explains LeGant. "The fourth dimension is the in-between world where lost souls go if they are disconnected from the Supreme Being or confused. For example, someone who has died and is in resistance toward leaving their family and moving on will be in this dimension."

The fourth dimension, which intersects our world, is home to a lot of beings, which are energy life forms that could also be called spirits. There's a wide spectrum of beings, whose nature depends upon their evolution, LeGant says. "Some are just observers, just watching and not interfering, some are very nice, helpful healers, and some are very destructive, harmful, negative beings that will lead people into mental illness, from suicide to depression to schizophrenia." They lead people into many other places as well. There's a being for almost everything, according to LeGant, and the influence of their dark energy is responsible for the negative state of the world.

There are beings that feed on sexual crime, on war, on negative thoughts, on control, on punishment, and on specific kinds of illness. Although the beings present depend entirely upon the individual, the general category of beings involved in addiction are "drug beings that thrive on the power they get from forcing someone to be addicted," explains LeGant. "The beings are very vicious when it comes to addiction," meaning that the messages they communicate to their hosts are particularly destructive.

Many of the thoughts and emotions that people with mental disorders, including addiction, experience have a lot to do with the beings in their space, says LeGant. Whether we are aware of it or not, we all are telepathic, meaning we can pick up on others' thoughts. This telepathic "wiring" is the source of the transmittal of thoughts. For example, you might have started on a recovery program or made a resolution to give up the substance to which you are addicted, and then you get this foreign thought telling you, "You can't do this, you'll fail, it's not going to work, it's hopeless, it's useless." That is the being in your space talking to you. It is also the urgings of the beings that prompt people to go out and obtain the drug or get up and pour a drink, even though they have resolved to quit or don't even want the substance at that moment.

"If it's a really nasty being, like a 'suicide being,' it will say, 'It's so hopeless, you may as well kill yourself, that's what you need to do,' and then the person is in so much pain that that's what ends up happening," says LeGant. "Those thoughts can be very intense and quite overwhelming."

The problem is that most people don't realize that these are *not* their thoughts, and they think that this is how they feel. People who are not developed clairvoyantly can't see the negative energy, so it is able to influence them and create confusion and angst. Influence by a being is often the case in people who go from doctor to doctor or other healer looking for a solution to their problem, to no avail. "What they need is someone to help them move the beings out of their space," which is what a spiritual healer such as LeGant does. The proviso for addiction, however, is that the person must have made the decision to stop using their substance of choice. Without that, moving the foreign beings out of that individual's energy field will produce only temporary benefit.

In addition, says LeGant, "withdrawal is not only from the chemical coming out of the brain and body, although that's certainly a factor, but the cravings, agitation, and other symptoms of withdrawal from a substance are also from the beings." When a person stops using, it threatens the beings' occupation of the person's space, he explains. They contribute to the withdrawal sensations to try to get the person to use again.

Pain Ridges and Core Pictures

In order to attach to people, the beings need something to anchor into. That something is pain, in the form of pain ridges and core pictures within people, LeGant explains.

Pain ridges are energy blockages in the body that are created during traumatic experiences. The pain associated with that trauma is stored in the body as a block of emotional energy, a pain ridge. "The beings plug into those pain ridges, into that old emotional energy, and it's like twisting a knife in someone's back," says LeGant. "They stimulate the old energies so the person continues to experience or sits in an old emotion that has nothing to do with what's going on in present time."

Beings also attach to what are called core pictures. These are made up of the emotions, thoughts, and sensory information associated with a trauma and are stored in the subconscious. The core pictures provide another anchor for beings that feed on that type of energy. The beings then keep that energy strong, active, and stimulated, or "lit up," as LeGant refers to it—like a bright spotlight on a picture.

Naturally, the content of core pictures is unique to each individual, but, as with the beings that are present, LeGant has seen common themes to the core pictures in clients with addiction problems. In general, the pictures tend to be those of invalidation and punishment. "The pictures are pain. They are living their core pictures, and that is why they are using." People with addictions typically have core pictures that teach them to use drugs to handle physical, psychological, or emotional pain. "It may be that they had addicted parents who gave them the message that when they feel pain, they need to get drunk or use drugs to numb it." Other common categories in addiction are victim pictures and apathy pictures.

Some of the pain ridges and core pictures are from past lifetimes and are often the result of past-life suicides, states LeGant. Suicide beings stimulate these past-life death ridges (the pain ridges having to do with one's death in a past life) and pictures, which contain the thoughts, emotions, and concepts of that long-ago moment of suicide. The body is always in present time, however, so it experiences the replaying of this pain as though it were happening now. "When the body gets stuck in a death picture, it will feel like it's dying," says LeGant. "It will experience what went on in that lifetime, and there's no rational explanation for where that emotion or that fear is coming from."

Again, drugs or alcohol will numb people to the painful reenactment of their core pictures, but the pictures and the associated pain are still there.

For psychics, attuned as they are to nonphysical forces and the spirit realm, the existence of past lives is a working, empirical reality. For those who are not as in tune with their psychic abilities, the concept of past lives may arouse skepticism. It is not necessary to believe in this, however, in order to be healed psychically. Regardless of one's conceptual model, the healing will clear the energies and pictures that are contributing to addiction or interfering in a person's optimal functioning in other ways.

Spiritual Healing

LeGant prefers to call what he does "spiritual healing" rather than "psychic healing" because the former is a more accurate description of what he is in fact doing, which is clearing the blockages to a person's connection to Spirit. He refers to this higher power as "the Supreme Being," which reflects its primacy over all the destructive beings that can occupy your energy field. A strong connection to the Supreme Being (God) is your best protection against the negative beings, which cannot thrive in an atmosphere of Light.

Spiritual healing involves eliminating the core pictures, dissolving the pain ridges, and removing all the negative beings from the person's energy field, says LeGant. Again, the content of all of this is unique to the individual, so the healing is never the same from one person to the next. In a session, LeGant and the client sit across from each other in comfortable chairs. To do his work, he goes into a light trance and, with eyes closed, "reads" what is happening in the client and sets about clearing the energy. Clients can choose to close their eyes or not during the process. By its very nature, psychic work does not require the client to be present. Spiritual healing can also be done long distance over the phone, which is how LeGant and many of his colleagues work most of the time.

The first week after the first session is usually very intense, LeGant notes. He calls this a growth period, which is somewhat like the "healing crisis" well known to natural medicine practitioners. "The core pictures are like the keystones in an arch. When you pull the keystones out, a lot of stuff starts falling apart. Some people have built their life on their pain. You go in and take out that foundation, and everything starts to go into flux; they redefine their reality. In the process of that, things die, and the person can feel like they're dying or like things are falling apart.

"After a week it starts to lighten up. After two weeks, you start to notice the joy underneath. It starts to come in and replace the pain with more lightness. If someone's in a crisis with their growth period, I just let them know that they can contact me. Usually they just need reassurance that it's normal. They don't need me to do anything."

In the case of addiction, LeGant states that he can remove the foreign energies and clear the blockages, but, as noted previously, unless people have made the decision to end their substance abuse, it will only be of temporary benefit. Most of his clients who suffer from addiction come to him for psychic insight into another problem they're having and say nothing about their substance abuse. But "addiction energy" is usually apparent to psychic vision, says LeGant, and he soon discovers it as he looks for the cause of the client's stated problem.

At that point, he gives the client a psychic acknowledgment of the addiction issue, "a clear, defined 'hello' on what's happening." The "hello" is communication on a soul level—LeGant's spirit saying to the client's spirit that there is a problem with addiction. He also communicates this message on a verbal level, saying it aloud to the person. It's then up to the client what he or she decides to do with that information. In some cases, the person already knows and may be trying to deal with it. In other cases, the person has not faced the problem, and the "hello" can help them do that.

For long-term users who are deeply in denial, the spirit-to-spirit communication doesn't accomplish much. "They have to make the decision," says LeGant. "I can't do it for them." For these clients, he doesn't do much healing work on the drug or alcohol energy because it will only be undone later when the person uses substances again. LeGant focuses instead on discharging the pain from the pictures the person is carrying.

Spiritual healing is not the passive process for the client that people typically associate with psychic readings. While LeGant "reads" the person and does the clearing needed for the person to move toward health, spiritual healing "has to do with a person's willingness to heal themselves, too," he says. "A lot of times people come to me wanting to dump their problems in my lap for me to solve them. But that's not what I do. I give them a 'hello' and clarity on what's going on. I give them information on the next steps that they can take to get what they want. I can move out a layer of blocks and obstacles that are in the way. But those are just blocks and obstacles. I can help make it easier for them, but they still need to make the choice to get well."

In the case of addiction, LeGant has found that many people are "scared to let go of their addictive energies and the depressions that go with them. People have to make a choice to get through something, and they may not be choosing that."

It is also necessary for people to learn how to handle their sensitivity, so they will not go back to absorbing foreign energies, says LeGant.

More specifically, his message is that you need to learn how to "be senior to energy" and how to define your own reality. This means not letting the beings or other people's energy determine your reality. In his Psychic School courses, LeGant teaches people how to accomplish this.

The following two cases illustrate how spiritual or psychic healing can be used with addiction. The case of Cecily is a fascinating and tragic depiction of how someone can use psychic clearing to keep them going but, without the commitment to healing, full recovery cannot occur. The case illustrates the role of pain in alcoholism and the great lengths to which people will go to avoid that pain. The case of David illustrates the large part that acknowledgment of a person's sensitivity and clairvoyance can play in ending addiction.

 There are many psychic healers, but not all work in the way described in this chapter. In addition to Leon LeGant (see the appendix for contact information for him and the Psychic School), graduates of the Berkeley Psychic Institute, of which LeGant is one, use some of these techniques (Berkeley Psychic Institute, Berkeley, CA; tel: 510-548-8020; website: www.berkeleypsychic.com). Lisa French, one of LeGant's teachers, also does psychic healings as described in this chapter and runs the Clairvoyant Center of Hawaii. For Lisa French, tel: 808-323-3199; website: www.magicisle.com/reading.htm. For the Clairvoyant Center, tel: 808-323-9699; website: www.clairvoyanthawaii.org.

Cecily: Running from Pain

Cecily, who was in her mid-forties, drank her way through a clairvoyant development program, as she had drunk her way through everything her whole adult life. Every night she drank a large bottle of wine, and every morning she used the psychic clearing techniques she had learned to "detoxify" or clear the effects of the alcohol she had ingested the night before. You could say that this was her own harm reduction program.

At one point, other people in the clairvoyant program, including LeGant, did psychic healing of her home to remove from it the influence of foreign energies. "There was a door in the house that she did not want us to open," he recalls. "We did anyway and found a closet stacked full of empty wine bottles. She was of course very embarrassed about that."

Along with her drinking, emotional drama was a way of life for Cecily. She spent a lot of time crying over her problems. In addition to the psychic clearings she did on herself, other people in the clairvoyant program, including LeGant, did clearings on her, but neither her problems nor her pain went away. Looking back on it, LeGant now sees that the reason was that "she would not choose to let go of the pain. She had the tools herself for dealing with it, for clearing it out of her, but she did not choose to do so." Ironically, as hard as she was running from the pain by trying to numb it with alcohol, she was also "sitting in the pain," staying in it and even identifying with it, as evidenced by her continual emotional dramas. But crying over her pain without facing its source was as ineffective as alcohol in releasing her from its bondage.

LeGant acknowledges how difficult it often is for us to face our pain. In the psychic clearing he does on himself, he sometimes encounters "a layer of pictures that I need to look directly at. I'll resist it for a month; I won't go into that space because it's charged for me, it's my pain pictures. It takes a little while of getting sick of it until I finally sit down and deal with it." Avoiding the pain is actually more painful than dealing with it, he observes. The clearing is easy to do and it's not an ordeal, but "there's still that unconscious mechanism of running away from pain, doing anything to avoid it, to not look at it. We all have certain levels of programming around that."

In recalling what he observed when he worked on Cecily, LeGant says, "I saw pain pictures, and I saw her numbing out her pain pictures and not wanting to deal with them. I also saw that she was not able to receive the information she was getting in the clairvoyant program because she wasn't in her body during her training." She removed a fair amount of her consciousness from her body so she could be free of the pain. In psychic terms, this meant she was hovering just above her head, leaving her body somewhat unattended.

"She was always detoxing, constantly cleaning out layers of alcohol that she had put in her body the night before, so she wasn't progressing," LeGant adds. "She needed to expose the pain underneath, so she could clear it out, but she never gave herself the opportunity to do that."

LeGant notes that Cecily's story, aside from the psychic training aspect, is not unusual among people who have been abusing substances for a long time. "For most of the people that I look at who are older and have been hooked into the drug game or the alcohol game for years, it's very difficult for them to get out of it. They're so used to it. It's their way of life."

People in their twenties, on the other hand, have typically not become so hooked into or adapted to addiction as a lifestyle. LeGant cites this as the reason why his success rate is so good with substance abusers in this age group. "My success rate is not 100 percent because it's still a free-will choice, but it's very high."

In LeGant's experience, the major obstacle to recovery is the choice to quit. But once people have made that decision, "they can go through the detox, do what they need to do, no matter how painful or uncomfortable it is, to get out of the game." He views relapse as a choice as well. "I don't believe in victims. Everyone makes choices, and they are responsible for what happens in their life. Good or bad, conscious or unconscious, they created it."

In the following case, David was heading for a life of addiction, but fortunately something sent him to LeGant when he still had a chance to turn things around.

David: *Every Drug There Was*

When David, 20, came to LeGant, he didn't say anything about why he was there or what he wanted. "He didn't say a word except his name when he sat down," recalls LeGant. As soon as LeGant started the reading, he saw massive drug use, of all kinds. There were holes in his brain from ecstasy, the sticky "numbed-out" energy found with habitual marijuana use, and traces of auric damage from everything from hallucinogens to heroin.

Later, David told him that he had started using drugs when he was 15 and went the opposite direction from what most people do. He began with the heaviest drugs and worked his way back to what are considered lighter drugs. He did everything—heroin, crack, cocaine, speed, hallucinogens, and marijuana.

When he came to LeGant, he was smoking marijuana every day and frequently taking ecstasy, as he often went to raves. "He would have done anything that crossed his path at that time, but what he was hooked on were the ecstasy and the pot."

"The ecstasy was the most damaging," recalls LeGant. "When someone has abused ecstasy to the point where there are holes in the brain, it becomes a chronic illness in and of itself." In David's case, this manifested as "tics in his mannerisms, how he held himself, and how he spoke. I don't mean slurred speech, but it was something like that, kind of a nervous speech pattern." He was also severely depressed and had been for a long time.

In addition to the drug damage that LeGant saw immediately upon beginning the reading, he saw

People in their twenties have typically not become so hooked into or adapted to addiction as a lifestyle as older people have. LeGant cites this as the reason why his success rate is so good with substance abusers in this age group. "My success rate is not 100 percent because it's still a free-will choice, but it's very high."

that David was one of those "genetic psychics" with a highly developed pineal gland. This translated into high sensitivity, which David didn't know how to control or handle, so he used drugs to numb it out. His ultrasensitivity was compounded by the fact that because he was so clairvoyant, he was perceived and saw himself as being very different from other people. Having a unique perspective is especially painful in adolescence, when everyone is trying to fit in. David's way of looking at the world made it hard for him to relate to the game-playing and the cliques at school. He couldn't fit in and didn't know how to relate.

Drugs did two things for David, says LeGant. They gave him a way of relating to everybody else and also got him out of his pain. By the time he came to LeGant, David had been taking one drug or another for five years.

Despite his heavy substance abuse, it was actually easy to get David off drugs. "All he really needed was a 'hello,'" LeGant recalls. "He needed to be validated that he is a unique soul and that he is clairvoyant. Most people are thirsty for psychic 'hellos'—your spirit telepathically acknowledging and greeting their spirit. Not many people on the planet know how to do this. Sometimes you give someone that spirit-to-spirit hello, and they get validated for the first time, everything grounds and stabilizes, and they start to feel good about themselves."

This was the case with David. "Once he understood what his path is and why he is here, he had enough will of his own to get out of the game." He stopped doing drugs after his first session with LeGant.

There were layers of healing that needed to be done after that, however, and they couldn't be done all at once because David could only handle so much at one time. One layer was repairing the extensive damage done by the drugs. In addition, LeGant had to remove and neutralize the effect of the drug wiring in David's brain and restore the energy flow in his organs, chakra system, and aura and other areas of drug damage.

With this work, David's tics and odd speech pattern went away. The reversal of the drug damage is not complete, but LeGant taught David how to do it himself, and he is still working on it. "It takes a while to get all that drug energy out," LeGant explains. "It took a while to get it in there, and it takes a while to get it out."

Another layer of healing involved clearing the foreign energies from David's energy field. In his case, there were a lot of "fear beings" feeding on his fears about feeling so disconnected and different.

Clearing David's core pain pictures was an especially crucial phase of the treatment. While his severe depression lessened after the first session, it took clearing his core pictures to resolve it completely. Many of his pain pictures involved feeling alienated or feeling abandoned. The latter was the result of his father leaving his family and "jerking them around" for years afterward. David also felt responsible for what happened to other people, personalized events around him, and "trashed himself" for everything, which built more levels of pain on top of the old pain pictures.

David is a good example of the combination of psychic sensitivity and a lot of pain being a setup for substance abuse. "Not knowing who he was and not being on his path were a big part of the addiction as well," observes LeGant. "Once he understood who he was and what he was doing here, it shifted everything around for him."

So why did David go for a psychic healing in the midst of his drug haze? LeGant's answer is that "the Supreme Being plopped him in front of me because of his path. That's a personal thing between a person and the Supreme Being. The Supreme Being was getting him out of the drug game so he could do what he was supposed to do, which was to develop his clairvoyance. The Supreme Being will use whoever and whatever to bring about what needs to happen. Sometimes the Supreme Being gives a person the answer to their prayers directly. Sometimes it comes through something on TV. Sometimes, some person crosses their path. In this case, the Supreme Being knew I had the information to help this person."

Having found the help he needed, it has now been three years since David stopped taking drugs, and he has had no relapses. Since receiving his "psychic hello," he has been developing his clairvoyance and has learned psychic tools for managing and clearing pain, so he no longer has a need for drugs. Now he's helping other people with addiction problems look at the energetic and pain issues behind their substance abuse and work toward healing the damage.

Conclusion

This book has provided you with a comprehensive and practical approach to ending your addictions. As you learned, the imbalances that can contribute to addiction range from nutritional deficiencies and allergies to energy disturbances and psychospiritual issues. Correcting these factors through the therapies detailed in this book or other methods has a dual purpose. As the imbalances underlying addiction can produce other symptoms and conditions, restoring balance on all levels is both an addiction recovery measure and good preventive medicine.

While all of us have to take responsibility for our own recovery, the fact that addiction is an epidemic around the world indicates that forces beyond the individual are operational. To end the epidemic, we need to discover the physical, environmental, social, and political conditions that are driving so many people to escape through drugs, alcohol, and other substances and activities. Is it worldwide environmental degradation that is destroying our health? Is it the social isolation and spiritual vacuum of twenty-first century life? Is it cultural factors that promote stimulation-seeking and consumption? Is it the economic conditions that make life untenable for most of the world's population?

The triple epidemic of addiction, depression, and anxiety, as well as the increase in a wide range of other disorders, is sending us a strong message: we better find the answers and we better do it soon, as there is no indication that our health crisis is getting anything but worse.

It is to be hoped that as more people find their way out of addiction through treatments such as those described in this book, they can bring their unique perspective to a broader analysis of the addiction epidemic and the search for global solutions. But it is up to all of us to heed the message of our current health crisis. With the state of the environment and the existence of worldwide medical policies, health is no longer an individual issue. We all have to take responsibility for the addictions afflicting so many of us.

Appendix
Resources

Practitioners in This Book

Johannes Beckmann, M.D.
E-mail: johannes_bbb@hotmail.com
Dr. Beckmann is a general practitioner and master of psychosomatic medicine (a European degree and medical specialty). His private practice in Palma de Mallorca, Spain, integrates biological medicine, a psychological approach to illness, and body-work therapy.

Ira J. Golchehreh, L.Ac., O.M.D.
2175-D Francisco Blvd.
San Rafael, CA 94901
Tel: (415) 485-4411
Licensed as an acupuncturist, doctor of oriental medicine, doctor of alternative medicine, and qualified medical evaluator (Q.M.E.) for the State of California, Dr. Golchehreh runs a general practice specializing in internal and external disorders, pain-related disorders, and sports/orthopedic medicine.

William M. Hitt, Dr. of Medicine and Surgery
William Hitt Center
Ave Paseo Tijuana 406, Suite 403

Tijuana, B.C. Mexico 22310
U.S. mailing address:
P.O. Box 434357
San Diego, CA 92143-4357
Tel: (888) 671-9849
Website: www.williamhittcenter.com
E-mail: wmhitt@williamhittcenter.com

Dr. Hitt, a researcher in immunocytopharmacology, developed Neurotransmitter Restoration (NTR), which involves the intravenous administration of amino acids, vitamins, and minerals. NTR is the therapeutic modality used at the ten-day residential treatment program for addiction at the William Hitt Center. The center's areas of specialty are addiction, immunology, and allergies.

Patricia Kaminski
Flower Essence Society
P.O. Box 459
Nevada City, CA 95959
Tel: (800) 736-9222 (U.S. and Canada) or (530) 265-9163
Fax: (530) 265-0584
E-mail: pkaminski@flowersociety.org
Website: www.flowersociety.org

Patricia Kaminski is an herbalist, flower essence therapist, co-director of the Flower Essence Society, author of *Flowers That Heal*, and coauthor of *Flower Essence Repertory*.

The Flower Essence Society is an international membership organization of health practitioners, researchers, students, and others interested in deepening knowledge of flower essence therapy. FES is devoted to research and education, and offers training and certification programs, and publications. The Society also provides a free networking service for finding a practitioner in your area.

Dietrich Klinghardt, M.D., Ph.D.
1200 112th Ave. NE, Suite A100
Bellevue, WA 98004
Tel: (425) 688-8818

Dr. Klinghardt specializes in Neural Therapy, Applied Psychoneurobiology, and Family Systems Therapy, which addresses the transgenerational energy legacies at the root of illness.

Rev. Leon S. LeGant
The Psychic School
Tel: (800) 951-8042
E-mail: leon@psychicschool.com
Website: www.psychicschool.com

LeGant is a psychic clairvoyant, spiritual healer, and executive director of the Psychic School, a nonprofit organization dedicated to the development of psychic abilities, spiritual awareness, and self-healing. The School offers readings, classes, retreats, short- and long-term training programs, and long-distance spiritual education.

Devi S. Nambudripad, M.D., D.C., L.Ac., Ph.D.
Pain Clinic
6714 Beach Blvd.
[Nambudripad Allergy Research Foundation
6732 Beach Blvd.]
Buena Park, CA 90621
Tel: (714) 523-8900
Website: www.naet.com

The Pain Clinic treats various pain and allergy disorders using NAET (Nambudripad's Allergy Elimination Techniques), acupuncture, and chiropractic. The Allergy Research Foundation is a nonprofit organization devoted to conducting clinical trials and studies on NAET and educating the public and professionals alike. Dr. Nambudripad is the author of numerous books, including *Say Good-Bye to Illness*.

Tony Roffers, Ph.D.
3542 Fruitvale Ave., Suite #218
Oakland, CA 94602-2327
Tel: (510) 531-6730
E-mail: tonyroffers@earthlink.net

Dr. Roffers is a licensed psychologist whose private practice with adult clients emphasizes Thought Field Therapy and Seemorg Matrix work for a wide variety of problems including addiction, anxiety, panic disorder, PTSD, depression, and food and inhalant sensitivities.

Julia Ross, M.A., Executive Director
Recovery Systems
147 Lomita Dr., Suite D
Mill Valley, CA 94941
Tel: (415) 383-3611 x2
Websites: www.dietcure.com and www.moodcure.com

Ross, a pioneer in the field of nutritional psychology and author of *The Mood Cure* and *The Diet Cure,* has 25 years of experience directing programs that address mood problems, addiction, and eating disorders. Her clinic, Recovery Systems, provides psychological and nutritional assessments, ongoing nutritional therapy, and holistic medical consultation. For more about her work with alcohol and drug addiction, see her book *The Mood Cure.* For more on her work with carbohydrate addiction, see her book *The Diet Cure.*

Recommended Reading

In addition to the books by the practitioners above, the following are recommended:

Blum, Kenneth, Ph.D., with James E. Payne. *Alcohol and the Addictive Brain.* New York: Free Press, 1991.

Callahan, Roger J., Ph.D. *The Anxiety-Addiction Connection: Eliminate Your Addictive Urges with Thought Field Therapy.* Indian Wells, CA: Roger J. Callahan, Ph.D., 1995. Available from: The Callahan Techniques, La Quinta, CA; (760) 564-1008.

Callahan, Roger J., Ph.D. *Stop Smoking Now!* The Callahan Techniques, 1987. Available from: The Callahan Techniques, La Quinta, CA; (760) 564-1008.

Grof, Christina. *The Thirst for Wholeness: Attachment, Addiction, and the Spiritual Path.* San Francisco, CA: HarperSanFrancisco, 1993.

Kasl, Charlotte Davis, Ph.D., *Women, Sex, and Addiction.* New York: Harper & Row, 1989.

Larson, Joan Mathews, Ph.D. *Seven Weeks to Sobriety: The Proven Program to Fight Alcoholism through Nutrition.* New York: Ballantine Wellspring, 1997.

Milam, James R., Ph.D., and Katherine Ketcham. *Under the Influence: A Guide to the Myths and Realities of Alcoholism.* New York: Bantam, 1981.

Phelps, Janice Keller, M.D., and Alan E. Nourse, M.D. *The Hidden Addiction and How to Get Free.* New York: Little, Brown, 1986.

Endnotes

Introduction

1. Anne Geller, M.D., "Common Addictions," *Clinic Symposia* 48:1 (1996): 2.

2. Barbara Yoder, *The Recovery Resource Book* (New York: Fireside/Simon & Schuster, 1990): 143.

3. Institute for Health Policy, Brandeis University, "Substance Abuse: The Nation's Number One Health Problem," 2001. Cited in "Alcoholism and Drug Dependence Are America's Number One Health Problem," on the website of the National Council on Alcoholism and Drug Dependence (NCADD): www.ncadd.org/facts/numberoneprob.html.

4. Anne Geller, M.D., "Common Addictions," 2.

5. J. Madeleine Nash, "Addicted," *Time Australia* (May 5, 1997).

6. "Sobering Facts on the Dangers of Alcohol," *NY Newsday* (April 24, 2002).

7. Michael McCarthy, "Prop 36 Prospects," *Pacific Sun* (March 7–13, 2001): 14.

8. Martin Rickler, Ph.D., "Acupuncture and Drug Treatment Literature Review: 1993," available on the Internet at www.crxs.com/Drug_Treatment.html.

9. Jean M. Twenge, "The Age of Anxiety? Birth Cohort Change in Anxiety and Neuroticism, 1952–1993," *Journal of Personality and Social Psychology* 79:6 (December 2000): 1007–21; available on the Internet at www.apa.org/journals/psp/psp7961007.html#c25s. NAMI, "Anxiety Disorders," available on the Internet at the NAMI website:

www.nami.org; or contact NAMI (National Alliance for the Mentally Ill), Colonial Place Three, 2107 Wilson Blvd., Suite 300, Alexandria, VA 22201-3042; tel: (888) 999-NAMI (6264) or (703) 524-7600.

10. NAMI, "Anxiety Disorders," available on the Internet at the NAMI website: www.nami.org.

11. P. Stokes and A. Holtz, "Fluoxetine tenth anniversary update: the progress continues," *Clinical Therapeutics* 19:5 (1997): 1135–250.

12. C. Murray and A. Lopez, eds., *The Global Burden of Disease: A Comprehensive Assessment of Mortality and Disability from Diseases, Injuries, and Risk Factors in 1990 and Projected to 2020* (Cambridge: Harvard University Press, 1996).

13. Lauran Neergaard, "Agency's Study Seeks Alcoholism Cure," *San Francisco Chronicle* (April 10, 2001): A7. Joan Mathews Larson, Ph.D., *Seven Weeks to Sobriety: The Proven Program to Fight Alcoholism through Nutrition* (New York: Ballantine Wellspring, 1997): 8.

14. Stanton Peele, Ph.D., and Archie Brodsky, *The Truth about Addiction and Recovery* (New York: Fireside/Simon & Schuster, 1991): 169; referring to George E. Vaillant, *The Natural History of Alcoholism: Causes, Patterns, and Paths to Recovery* (Cambridge, MA: Harvard University Press, 1983): 284.

15. Stanton Peele, Ph.D., and Archie Brodsky, *The Truth about Addiction and Recovery* (New York: Fireside/Simon & Schuster, 1991): 32; referring to William R. Miller and Reid K. Hester, "The Effectiveness of Alcoholism Treatment: What Research Reveals," in W. R. Miller and N. K. Heather, eds., *Treating Addictive Behaviors: Processes of Change* (New York: Plenum, 1986): 136.

1: What Is Addiction and Who Suffers from It?

16. Terence T. Gorski and Merlene Miller, *Staying Sober: A Guide for Relapse Prevention* (Independence, MO: Herald House/Independence Press, 1986): 39.

17. Charlotte Davis Kasl, Ph.D., *Women, Sex, and Addiction* (New York: Harper & Row, 1989): 19.

18. Craig Nakken, *The Addictive Personality: Understanding the Addictive Process and Compulsive Behavior* (Center City, MN: Hazelden Information and Educational Services, 1996): 2.

19. Ibid., 27.

20. "Am I an Addict?" Narcotics Anonymous World Services literature, 1988; available on the Internet at www.na.org/ips/eng/IP7.htm.

21. Stanton Peele, Ph.D., and Archie Brodsky, *The Truth about Addiction and Recovery* (New York: Fireside/Simon & Schuster, 1991): 22.

22. Craig Nakken, *The Addictive Personality*, 13. The Hazelden treatment model (known as the Minnesota Model) is based on Twelve-Step principles.

23. Statement by researcher Nora Volkow, M.D., of the Brookhaven National Laboratory in New York. Cited in J. Madeleine Nash, "Addicted," *Time Australia* (May 5, 1997).

24. Katie Evans, C.A.D.C., and J. Michael Sullivan, Ph.D., *Dual Diagnosis Series: Understanding Major Anxiety Disorders and Addiction* (Center City, MN: Hazelden, 1991): 6–7.

25. American Psychiatric Association, *DSM-IV-TR* (*Diagnostic and Statistical Manual of Mental Disorders, 4th Edition, Text Revision*), Washington, D.C.: American Psychiatric Association, 2000: 192.

26. Ibid., 197.

27. Ibid., 199.

28. Institute for Health Policy, Brandeis University, "Substance Abuse: The Nation's Number One Health Problem," 2001. Cited in "Alcoholism and Drug Dependence Are America's Number One Health Problem," on the website of the National Council on Alcoholism and Drug Dependence (NCADD): www.ncadd.org/facts/numberoneprob.html.

29. National Institute on Alcohol Abuse and Alcoholism (NIAAA), "Alcoholism: Getting the Facts," available on the Internet: www.niaaa.nih.gov/publications/booklet.htm.

30. "Doctors Failing to Help Addicts," *San Francisco Chronicle* (January 22, 2001).

31. Sandra Blakeslee, "Meth's Harm to Brain Worse Than Believed," *San Francisco Chronicle* (March 6, 2001): A9.

32. John Cloud, "The Lure of Ecstasy," *Time* (June 5, 2000): 64.

33. Institute for Health Policy, Brandeis University, "Substance Abuse: The Nation's Number One Health Problem," 2001. Cited in "Alcoholism and Drug Dependence Are America's Number One Health Problem," on the website of the National Council on Alcoholism and Drug Dependence (NCADD): www.ncadd.org/facts/numberoneprob.html.

34. Ibid.

35. The National Drug Control Strategy, The White House, 1997. Cited in "Alcoholism and Drug Dependence Are America's Number One Health Problem," on the website of the National Council on Alcoholism and Drug Dependence (NCADD): www.ncadd.org/facts/numberoneprob.html.

36. Janice Keller Phelps, M.D., and Alan E. Nourse, M.D., *The Hidden Addiction and How to Get Free* (New York: Little, Brown, 1986): 39.

37. Martin Rickler, Ph.D., "Acupuncture and Drug Treatment Literature Review: 1993," available on the Internet at www.crxs.com/Drug_Treatment.html.

38. Craig Nakken, *The Addictive Personality*, 3.

39. Janice Keller Phelps and Alan E. Nourse, *The Hidden Addiction and How to Get Free*, 5–6.

40. Institute for Health Policy, Brandeis University, "Substance Abuse: The Nation's Number One Health Problem," 2001. Cited in "Alcoholism and Drug Dependence Are America's Number One Health Problem," on the website of the National Council on Alcoholism and Drug Dependence (NCADD): www.ncadd.org/facts/numberoneprob.html.

41. National Institute on Alcohol Abuse and Alcoholism (NIAAA), "Alcoholism: Getting the Facts," available on the Internet: http://www.niaaa.nih.gov/publications/booklet.htm.

42. Stanton Peele, and Archie Brodsky, *The Truth about Addiction and Recovery*, 52.

43. Anne Geller, M.D., "Common Addictions," *Clinic Symposia* 48:1 (1996): 8–9. Barbara Yoder, *The Recovery Resource Book*, 42, 190.

44. Joan Mathews Larson, Ph.D., *Seven Weeks to Sobriety: The Proven Program to Fight Alcoholism through Nutrition* (New York: Ballantine Wellspring, 1997): 9.

45. Anne Geller, "Common Addictions," 2.

46. "Sobering Facts on the Dangers of Alcohol," *NY Newsday* (April 24, 2002).

47. Lauran Neergaard, "Agency's Study Seeks Alcoholism Cure," *San Francisco Chronicle* (April 10, 2001): A7.

48. "Doctors Failing to Help Addicts," *San Francisco Chronicle* (January 22, 2001).

49. Institute for Health Policy, Brandeis University, "Substance Abuse:

The Nation's Number One Health Problem," 2001. Cited in "Alcoholism and Drug Dependence Are America's Number One Health Problem," on the website of the National Council on Alcoholism and Drug Dependence (NCADD): www.ncadd.org/facts/numberoneprob.html.

50. Sandra Blakeslee, "Meth's Harm to Brain Worse Than Believed," A9.

51. John Cloud, "The Lure of Ecstasy," *Time* (June 5, 2000): 64.

52. Ibid.

53. Ibid.

54. Barbara Yoder, *The Recovery Resource Book* (New York: Fireside/Simon & Shuster, 1990): 184.

55. Karl Taro Greenfeld, "Speed Demons," *Time* (April 2, 2001): 39.

56. Sandra Blakeslee, "Meth's Harm to Brain Worse Than Believed," A9.

57. Karl Taro Greenfeld, "Speed Demons," 39.

58. Joseph Volpicelli, M.D., Ph.D., and Maia Szalavitz, *Recovery Options: The Complete Guide* (New York: John Wiley & Sons, 2000): 27.

59. Susan Greenfield, "Pot Really Can Blow Your Mind," *San Francisco Chronicle* (January 6, 2002).

60. National Institute on Drug Abuse (NIDA), "Information on Commonly Abused Drugs," available on the Internet at: www.nida.nih.gov/DrugsofAbuse.html.

61. Barbara Yoder, *The Recovery Resource Book,* 207.

62. Stanton Peele, and Archie Brodsky, *The Truth about Addiction and Recovery,* 76.

63. *DSM-IV-TR,* 481. Harold H. Bloomfield, *Healing Anxiety Naturally* (New York: Perennial Press, 1999): 38.

64. Muriel MacFarlane, R.N., M.A., *The Panic Attack, Anxiety, and Phobia Solutions Handbook* (Leucadia, CA: United Research Publishers, 1995): 251–2.

65. Harold H. Bloomfield, M.D., *Healing Anxiety Naturally,* 40.

66. Jerilyn Ross, *Triumph Over Fear: A Book of Help and Hope for People with Anxiety, Panic Attacks, and Phobias* (New York: Bantam Books, 1994): 265.

67. Thank you to Leah Garchik, *San Francisco Chronicle* columnist, for this tidbit.

68. Richard Corliss, "Who's Feeling No Pain?" *Time South Pacific* (March 19, 2001).

69. Ibid.

70. Anne Geller, "Common Addictions," 19.

71. Richard Corliss, "Who's Feeling No Pain?" *Time South Pacific* (March 19, 2001).

72. Santa Fe Rape Crisis Center, "When Drugs Are Used to Rape: Rohypnol and Drug-Facilitated Rape," article available on the Internet at: www.sfrcc.org/drugs.html.

73. Donald R. Wesson, M.D., David E. Smith, M.D., and Sarah Calhoun, M.P.H., "Rohypnol & Other Benzodiazepines of Abuse in South Texas," article posted on the Internet at www.hafci.org/research/index.html.

74. Ibid.

75. Charles Gant, M.D., Ph.D., "A Natural Answer to ADHD," *Healthy and Natural Journal* 7:4, 7:35 (August 1, 2000): 66–68, 70–71.

76. Jule Klotter, "Ritalin—An Addict's Story," *Townsend Letter for Doctors and Patients* 205/206 (August 1, 2000): 20.

77. Anne Geller, "Common Addictions," 19.

78. Elizabeth Wurtzel, "Adventures in Ritalin," *New York Times* (April 1, 2000). Cited in Jule Klotter, "Ritalin—An Addict's Story," *Townsend Letter for Doctors and Patients* 205/206 (August 1, 2000): 20.

79. Ibid.

80. J. Madeleine Nash, "Addicted," *Time Australia* (May 5, 1997).

81. Anne Geller, "Common Addictions," 25.

82. Stanton Peele, and Archie Brodsky, *The Truth about Addiction and Recovery,* 96.

83. Barbara Yoder, *The Recovery Resource Book*, 126, 127.

84. Anne Geller, "Common Addictions," 2.

85. Jane Ganahl, "The Softer Side of Addiction," *San Francisco Chronicle* (May 18, 2003): E1.

86. Stanton Peele and Archie Brodsky, *The Truth about Addiction and Recovery*, 116.

87. Ellen Ruppel Shell, "It's Not the Carbs, Stupid," *Newsweek* (August 5, 2002): 41.

88. Personal communication with author, 2003.

89. "Internet Addiction No Laughing Matter," *Spectrum: The Holistic Health News Digest* 70 (April 30, 2000): 28.

90. "Researchers Assess Addiction to Internet," *International Council for Health Freedom Newsletter* 4:2 (June 30, 2000): 48.

91. Anne Geller, "Common Addictions," 2. Stanton Peele, and Archie Brodsky, *The Truth about Addiction and Recovery,* 100.

92. Michael Herkov, Ph.D., Mark S. Gold, M.D., and Drew W. Edwards, M.S., "Treatment for Sexual Addiction," University of Florida Brain Institute (February 29, 2000); available on the Internet at: http://open-mind.org/News/SLA/4c.htm.

93. Steve K. Dubrow-Eichel, Ph.D., "Hypnosis in Client-Centered Addictions Counseling: Evolution of a Paradigm," paper presented to the 1997 Annual Conference of the American Psychological Association; available on the internet at: http://users.snip.net/~drsteve/Articles/APA_1997.html.

94. Patrick Carnes, Ph.D., *Don't Call It Love: Recovery from Sexual Addiction* (New York: Bantam, 1991): 107.

95. Ibid.

96. Joseph Volpicelli, and Maia Szalavitz, *Recovery Options,* 25.

97. Ibid., 250.

98. NIMH, "Anxiety Disorders," National Institute of Mental Health (NIH Publication No. 00-3879, reprinted 2000); available on the Internet at: www.nimh.nih.gov/anxiety/anxiety.cfm. *DSM-IV-TR,* 435–6, 465–6.

99. John R. Marshall, M.D., *Social Phobia: From Shyness to Stage Fright* (New York: Basic Books, 1994): 152.

100. R. Reid Wilson, Ph.D., *Don't Panic: Taking Control of Anxiety Attacks* (New York: Perennial Press, 1996): 98.

101. J. P. Lepine, J. M. Chignon, and M. Teherani, "Suicide Attempts in Patients with Panic Disorder," *Archives of General Psychiatry* 50:2 (1993): 144–9. Cited in: Frank J. Ayd Jr., M.D., and Claudia Daileader, "The Correlation between Suicide and Panic Disorder," *Psychiatric Times* 17:9 (September 2000); available on the Internet at: www.psychiatrictimes.com/p000937.html.

102. Linda Schierse Leonard, *Witness to the Fire: Creativity and the Veil of Addiction* (Boston: Shambhala, 1990): xv–xvi.

103. Barbara Yoder, *The Recovery Resource Book,* 9.

104. James R. Milam, Ph.D., and Katherine Ketcham, *Under the Influence: A Guide to the Myths and Realities of Alcoholism* (New York: Bantam, 1981): 136.

105. Ibid., 142.

106. Kenneth Blum, Ph.D., with James E. Payne, *Alcohol and the Addictive Brain* (New York: Free Press, 1991): 237.

107. J. Madeleine Nash, "Addicted," *Time Australia* (May 5, 1997).

108. Ibid.

109. Anne Geller, "Common Addictions," 25.

110. E. C. Azmitia and P. M. Whitaker-Azmitia, "Awakening the Sleeping Giant: Anatomy and Plasticity of the Brain Serotonergic System," *Journal of Clinical Psychiatry* 52:12 suppl. (1991): 4–16. Cited in Joseph Glenmullen, M.D., *Prozac Backlash* (New York: Touchstone/Simon & Schuster, 2000): 16.

111. Julia Ross, M.A., *The Diet Cure* (New York: Penguin, 1999): 121.

112. Russell Jaffe, M.D., Ph.D., and Oscar Rogers Kruesi, M.D., "The Biochemical-Immunology Window: A Molecular View of Psychiatric Case Management," *Journal of Applied Nutrition* 44:2 (1992).

113. Julia Ross, M.A., *The Diet Cure*, 120.

114. Joseph Volpicelli, M.D., Ph.D., and Maia Szalavitz, *Recovery Options: The Complete Guide*, 145.

115. Henrick J. Harwood, "Societal Costs of Heroin Addiction," paper presented at the NIH Consensus Development Conference on Effective Medical Treatment of Heroin Addiction, November 17–19, 1997, Bethesda, MD.

116. Michael Herkov, Ph.D., Mark S. Gold, M.D., and Drew W. Edwards, M.S., "Treatment for Sexual Addiction," University of Florida Brain Institute (February 29, 2000); available on the Internet at: http://open-mind.org/News/SLA/4c.htm.

2: Causes, Contributors, and Influences

117. Joseph Volpicelli, M.D., Ph.D., and Maia Szalavitz, *Recovery Options: The Complete Guide* (New York: John Wiley & Sons, 2000): 10.

118. James R. Milam, Ph.D., and Katherine Ketcham, *Under the Influence: A Guide to the Myths and Realities of Alcoholism* (New York: Bantam, 1981): 31. Barbara Yoder, *The Recovery Resource Book* (New York: Fireside/Simon & Schuster, 1990): 32.

119. Stanton Peele and Archie Brodsky, *The Truth about Addiction and Recovery* (New York: Fireside/Simon & Schuster, 1991): 96.

120. Anne Geller, "Common Addictions," *Clinic Symposia* 48:1 (1996): 5.

121. Stanton Peele and Archie Brodsky, *The Truth about Addiction and Recovery,* 62.

122. Anne Geller, "Common Addictions," 11.

123. J. Madeleine Nash, "Addicted," *Time Australia* (May 5, 1997).

124. Kenneth Blum, Ph.D., with James E. Payne, *Alcohol and the Addictive Brain* (New York: Free Press, 1991): 237.

125. Information from the website of Kenneth Blum, Ph.D. (www.docbluminc.com). Kenneth Blum, Ph.D., with Julia Ross, M.A., et al., "Nutritional Gene Therapy: Natural Healing in Recovery," *Counselor Magazine: The Magazine for Addiction Professionals* (January/February 2001); available on the Internet at www.counselor magazine.com/display_article.asp?aid=Nutritional_Gene_Therapy. aspv.

126. Joan Mathews Larson, Ph.D., *Seven Weeks to Sobriety: The Proven Program to Fight Alcoholism through Nutrition* (New York: Ballantine Wellspring, 1997): 30.

127. Stephanie Marohn, *The Natural Medicine Guide to Autism* (Charlottesville, VA: Hampton Roads, 2002): 118.

128. Cindy R. Mogil, *Swallowing a Bitter Pill: How Prescription and Over-the-Counter Drug Abuse Is Ruining Lives—My Story* (Far Hills, NJ: New Horizon Press, 2001): 16.

129. Kenneth Blum, *Alcohol and the Addictive Brain,* 181.

130. Simone Gabbay, "Kicking Addiction," *Alive Magazine: Canadian Journal of Health and Nutrition* 216 (October 1, 2000): 34–35.

131. Janice Keller Phelps, M.D., and Alan E. Nourse, M.D., *The Hidden Addiction and How to Get Free* (New York: Little, Brown, 1986): 47.

132. Francis Hartigan, *Bill W.: A Biography of Alcoholics Anonymous Cofounder Bill Wilson* (New York: St. Martin's Press, 2000): 205–08.

133. "A Newcomer Asks," Alcoholics Anonymous literature, available on the Internet at: www.alcoholics-anonymous.org/default/en_about_aa.cfm?pageid=10.

134. Francis Hartigan, *Bill W.,* 206.

135. Kenneth Blum, *Alcohol and the Addictive Brain,* 211–12.

136. Anne Geller, "Common Addictions," 8. Joan Mathews Larson, Ph.D., *Seven Weeks to Sobriety,* 106, 110. Eva Edelman, *Natural Healing*

for Schizophrenia and Other Common Mental Disorders, 3d ed. (Eugene, OR: Borage Books, 2001): 86.

137. Linda Rector Page, N.D., Ph.D., *Healthy Healing* (Carmel Valley, CA: Healthy Healing Publications, 1997): 103.

138. James F. Balch, M.D., and Phyllis A. Balch, C.N.C., *Prescription for Nutritional Healing*, (Garden City Park, NY: Avery Publishing Group, 1990): 7.

139. Joan Mathews Larson, *Seven Weeks to Sobriety*, 104–05.

140. Janice Keller Phelps and Alan E. Nourse, *The Hidden Addiction*, 47.

141. Ibid., 51, 124.

142. Michael Lesser, M.D., *Nutrition and Vitamin Therapy* (New York: Bantam, 1981): 109–10.

143. Melvyn R. Werbach, M.D., *Nutritional Influences on Illness: A Sourcebook of Clinical Research* (Tarzana, CA: Third Line Press, 1994): 37-38. Michael Lesser, *Nutrition and Vitamin Therapy*, 109.

144. Stephanie Marohn, *The Natural Medicine Guide to Bipolar Disorder* (Charlottesville, VA: Hampton Roads, 2003): 108, 109.

145. Ibid., 109.

146. M. A. Crawford, A. G. Hassam, and P. A. Stevens, "Essential fatty acid requirements in pregnancy and lactation with special reference to brain development," *Progress in Lipid Research* 20 (1981): 31–40.

147. "Healing Mood Disorders with Essential Fatty Acids," *Doctors' Prescription for Healthy Living* 4:6, 1.

148. Joseph Volpicelli, and Maia Szalavitz, *Recovery Options*, 212.

149. Joan Mathews Larson, *Seven Weeks to Sobriety*, 109.

150. Ibid., 35–36.

151. Ibid., 35.

152. James R. Milam, Ph.D., and Katherine Ketcham, *Under the Influence: A Guide to the Myths and Realities of Alcoholism* (New York: Bantam, 1981): 154.

153. Joan Mathews Larson, *Seven Weeks to Sobriety*, 9, 123, 134.

154. Ibid., xvii.

155. Janice Keller Phelps, M.D., and Alan E. Nourse, M.D., *The Hidden Addiction and How to Get Free*, 8.

156. Joan Mathews Larson, *Seven Weeks to Sobriety*, 132.

157. Ibid., 41.

158. David L. Murphy, M.D., "Alcoholism: The Genetic Link," *Sober Times* (March 1988); cited in Barbara Yoder, *The Recovery Resource Book* (New York: Fireside/Simon & Schuster, 1990): 44.

159. Sherry A. Rogers, M.D., *Depression: Cured at Last!* (Sarasota, FL: SK Publishing, 1997): 460.

160. Allan Sachs, D.C., C.C.N., *The Authoritative Guide to Grapefruit Seed Extract* (Mendocino, CA: LifeRhythm, 1997): 58.

161. Sherry A. Rogers, *Depression,* 165–7.

162. Ibid., 166.

163. Jerilyn Ross, *Triumph Over Fear: A Book of Help and Hope for People with Anxiety, Panic Attacks, and Phobias* (New York: Bantam Books, 1994): 257.

164. Joan Mathews Larson, *Seven Weeks to Sobriety,* 41–42, 261.

165. Allan Sachs, *The Authoritative Guide,* 61.

166. Personal communication, 2001.

167. Syd Baumel, *Dealing with Depression Naturally* (Los Angeles: Keats Publishing, 2000): 12.

168. Anne Geller, "Common Addictions," 8.

169. Janice Keller Phelps, M.D., and Alan E. Nourse, M.D., *The Hidden Addiction and How to Get Free,* 27–28.

170. Joseph Glenmullen, M.D., *Prozac Backlash* (New York: Touchstone/Simon & Schuster, 2000): 340.

171. Joan Mathews Larson, *Seven Weeks to Sobriety,* 135.

172. Jennifer A. Phillips, "Thyroid Hormone Disorders," Cambridge Scientific Abstracts (released May 2001); available on the Internet at: www.csa.com/hottopics/thyroid/oview.html.

173. Ibid.

174. Suzanne Diamond, "Alleviating Addictions: Herbs That Help," *Healthy & Natural Journal* 6:5, Issue 30 (October 31, 1999): 101–03.

175. Burton Goldberg and the editors of *Alternative Medicine, Women's Health Series: 2* (Tiburon, CA: Future Medicine Publishing, 1998): 208–209.

176. Suzanne Diamond, "Alleviating Addictions: Herbs That Help," *Healthy & Natural Journal* 6:5, Issue 30 (October 31, 1999): 101–03.

177. Richard Leviton, *The Healthy Living Space* (Charlottesville, VA: Hampton Roads, 2001): 2.

178. "Doctors warn developmental disabilities epidemic from tox-

ins," *LDA (Learning Disabilities Association of America) Newsbriefs* 35:4 (July/August 2000): 3–5; executive summary from the report by the Greater Boston Physicians for Social Responsibility, *In Harm's Way: Toxic Threats to Child Development*, available at www.igc.org/psr/ihw.htm; for LDA, www.ldanatl.org.

179. Philip J. Landrigan, *Environmental Neurotoxicology* (Washington, D.C.: National Academy Press, 1992): 2; cited in Richard Leviton, *The Healthy Living Space*, 13.

180. Sherry A. Rogers, *Depression*, 94.

181. Joan Mathews Larson, *Seven Weeks to Sobriety*, 34.

182. John Foster, M.D., "Is Depression Natural in an Unnatural World?" *Well-Being Journal* (Spring 2001): 11; website: www.wellbeing journal.com.

183. Dietrich Klinghardt, M.D., Ph.D., "Amalgam/Mercury Detox as a Treatment for Chronic Viral, Bacterial, and Fungal Illnesses," lecture presented at the Annual Meeting of the International and American Academy of Clinical Nutrition, San Diego, CA, September 1996.

184. Morton Walker, D.P.M., *Elements of Danger: Protect Yourself against the Hazards of Modern Dentistry* (Charlottesville, VA: Hampton Roads, 2000): 138, 141.

185. Joseph Volpicelli, and Maia Szalavitz, *Recovery Options*, 238.

186. Lee Robins, Darlene Davis, and Donald Goodwin, "Drug Use in U.S. Army Enlisted Men in Vietnam: A Follow-Up on Their Return," *American Journal of Epidemiology* 99 (1974): 235–49.

187. James R. Milam, Ph.D., and Katherine Ketcham, *Under the Influence*, 155.

188. Rita Elkins, *Depression and Natural Medicine: A Nutritional Approach to Depression and Mood Swings* (Pleasant Grove, UT: Woodland Publishing, 1995): 138. Eva Edelman, *Natural Healing for Schizophrenia and Other Common Mental Disorders*, 85.

189. Rita Elkins, *Depression and Natural Medicine*, 138.

190. Eva Edelman, *Natural Healing*, 134.

191. Rita Elkins, *Depression and Natural Medicine*, 103. Eva Edelman, *Natural Healing*, 40.

192. Janice Keller Phelps, and Alan E. Nourse, *The Hidden Addiction and How to Get Free*, 110.

193. Stanton Peele, and Archie Brodsky, *The Truth about Addiction and Recovery,* 14.

3: The Biochemistry of Addiction: Amino Acids and NTR

194. Personal communication and Julia Ross, M.A., *The Diet Cure* (New York: Penguin, 1999): 15.

195. Julia Ross, *The Diet Cure,* 128.

196. Adapted from: Julia Ross, M.A., *The Mood Cure* (New York: Viking, 2002): 258–61.

197. Julia Ross, *The Diet Cure,* 120.

198. Cindy R. Mogil, *Swallowing a Bitter Pill: How Prescription and Over-the-Counter Drug Abuse Is Ruining Lives—My Story* (Far Hills, NJ: New Horizon Press, 2001): 4.

4: Allergies and Addiction: NAET

199. Devi S. Nambudripad, M.D., D.C., L.Ac., Ph.D., *Say Goodbye to Illness,* new & revised ed. (Buena Park, CA: Delta Publishing, 1999): 448.

200. Caroline Knapp, *Drinking: A Love Story* (New York: Dial Press, 1996): 456.

201. Ibid., 243.

202. Ibid., 457.

203. Devi S. Nambudripad, M.D., D.C., L.Ac., Ph.D., *Say Goodbye to Allergy-Related Autism* (Buena Park, CA: Delta Publishing, 1999): 32–47. Devi S. Nambudripad, *Say Goodbye to Illness,* 296.

204. Devi S. Nambudripad, *Say Goodbye to Illness,* xxii.

205. Personal communication with Dr. Nambudripad, 2001. Richard Leviton, "The Allergy-Free Body," *Alternative Medicine Digest* 6 (April 1995): 13.

206. Devi S. Nambudripad, *Say Goodbye to Illness,* xxiii.

207. Ibid., 147–8.

208. Richard Leviton, "The Allergy-Free Body," *Alternative Medicine Digest* 6 (April 1995): 8.

209. "New Evidence Points to Opioids," *Autism Research Review International* 5:4 (1991).

210. Paul Shattock, "Urinary Peptides and Associated Metabolites in the Urine of People with Autism Spectrum Disorders," syllabus

material for the main DAN! lecture at the DAN! (Defeat Autism Now!) 2000 Conference, in the conference booklet: 79–83; published by the Autism Research Institute in San Diego, CA (fax: 619-563-6840 or website: www.autism.com/ari). "New Evidence Points to Opioids," *Autism Research Review International* 5:4 (1991). A. J. Wakefield et al., "Ileal-Lymphoid-Nodular Hyperplasia, Non-Specific Colitis, and Pervasive Developmental Disorder in Children," *Lancet* 351 (February 28, 1998): 637–41.

211. C. Hallert et al., "Psychic Disturbances in Adult Coeliac Disease III. Reduced Central Monoamine Metabolism and Signs of Depression," *Scandinavian Journal of Gastroenterology* 17 (1982): 25–8.

212. Ron Hoggan, M.A., and James Braly, M.D., "How Modern Eating Habits May Contribute to Depression," available on the Internet at: http://depression.about.com/library/weekly/aa071299.htm.

213. See Depression: Causes (Food Allergies/Intolerances) at: www.yournutrition.co.uk/health_problems/depression_m.htm.

214. Devi S. Nambudripad, *Say Goodbye to Illness*, 33.

5: Energy Medicine I: Traditional Chinese Medicine

215. "NIH Consensus Conference: Acupuncture," *JAMA* 280:17 (November 4, 1998): 1518–24.

216. Martin Rickler, Ph.D., "Acupuncture and Drug Treatment Literature Review: 1993," available on the Internet at www.crxs.com/Drug_Treatment.html.

217. Ibid.

218. Dennis Wholey, *The Courage to Change* (Boston: Houghton Mifflin, 1984): 142.

6: Energy Medicine II: Flower Essence Therapy

219. Edward Bach and F .J. Wheeler, *The Bach Flower Remedies* (New Canaan, CT: Keats Publishing, 1977).

220. Patricia Kaminski and Richard Katz, *Flower Essence Repertory* (Nevada City, CA: Flower Essence Society, 1996): 5. Patricia Kaminski and Richard Katz, "Using Flower Essences: A Practical Overview," publication of the Flower Essence Society, Nevada City, CA, 1994.

221. Barbara Yoder, *The Recovery Resource Book* (New York: Fireside/Simon & Schuster, 1990): 7.

222. Patricia Kaminski and Richard Katz, *Flower Essence Repertory*, 3.

223. "The Flower Essence Society: Pioneering Research and Education in Flower Essence Therapy," booklet published by the Flower Essence Society, Nevada City, CA: 10.

224. Jeffrey Cram, Ph.D., "FES Launches a Major Multi-Site Scientific Study on Flower Essences and the Treatment of Depression," *Flower Essence Society Newsletter* (Spring 2000): 1.

225. Patricia Kaminski and Richard Katz, *Flower Essence Repertory*, 348.

226. Ibid., 402.

227. Ibid., 293, 302.

228. Ibid., 296

7: The Five Levels of Healing

229. Christina Grof, *The Thirst for Wholeness: Attachment, Addiction, and the Spiritual Path* (San Francisco, CA: HarperSan Francisco, 1993): 1, 15.

8: Energy, Trauma, and Spirit: TFT and Seemorg Matrix Work

230. Roger J. Callahan, Ph.D., *The Anxiety-Addiction Connection: Eliminate Your Addictive Urges with Thought Field Therapy* (Indian Wells, CA: Roger J. Callahan, Ph.D., 1995): 15. Available from: The Callahan Techniques, La Quinta, CA; (760) 564-1008.

231. Ibid., 7.

232. Ibid., 13.

233. Ibid., 7.

234. Ibid., 5.

235. Roger J. Callahan, Ph.D., *Tapping the Healer Within: Using Thought Field Therapy to Instantly Conquer Your Fears, Anxieties, and Emotional Distress* (Chicago: Contemporary Books, 2001): 12.

236. Roger J. Callahan, *The Anxiety-Addiction Connection*, 8.

237. Ibid., 9, 10.

238. Karl Taro Greenfeld, "Speed Demons," *Time* (April 2, 2001): 37, 38.

239. Nahoma Asha Clinton, L.C.S.W., Ph.D., "Seemorg Matrix Work, The Transpersonal Energy Psychotherapy," available on the Internet at www.matrixwork.org/tara.html.

240. Ibid.

241. Nahoma Asha Clinton, L.C.S.W., Ph.D., "The Story of SEEMORG," available on the Internet at www.seemorgmatrix.org/seemorg-story.html.

242. Nahoma Asha Clinton, L.C.S.W., Ph.D., "Redefining Trauma," available on the Internet at www.matrixwork.org/manual.htm.

243. Information from the website of the Albert Ellis Institute (Albert Ellis developed REBT) and Rational Emotive Behavior Therapy (REBT): www.rebt.org/.

9: Psychic Healing

244. Richard Leviton, *The Healthy Living Space* (Charlottesville, VA: Hampton Roads, 2001): 354–8.

245. Ibid., 362–3.

246. Ibid., 364.

247. Barbara Yoder, *The Recovery Resource Book* (New York: Fireside/Simon & Schuster, 1990): 7.

Index

About the Author

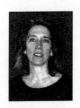

Stephanie Marohn has been writing since she was a child. Her adult writing background is extensive in both journalism and nonfiction trade books. In addition to *Natural Medicine First Aid Remedies* and the six books in the Healthy Mind Series (*The Natural Medicine Guide to Autism, The Natural Medicine Guide to Depression, The Natural Medicine Guide to Bipolar Depression, The Natural Medicine Guide to Addiction, The Natural Medicine Guide to Anxiety,* and *The Natural Medicine Guide to Schizophrenia*), she has published more than thirty articles in magazines and newspapers, written two novels and a feature film screenplay, and has had her work included in poetry, prayer, and travel writing anthologies.

Originally from Philadelphia, she has been a resident of the San Francisco Bay Area for over twenty years, and currently lives in Sonoma Country, north of the city.

Please visit www.stephaniemarohn.com for more information.

Hampton Roads Publishing Company

. . . for the evolving human spirit

Hampton Roads Publishing Company
publishes books on a variety of subjects,
including metaphysics, health,
visionary fiction, and other related topics.

For a copy of our latest catalog, call toll-free
(800) 766-8009, or send your name and address to:

Hampton Roads Publishing Company, Inc.
1125 Stoney Ridge Road
Charlottesville, VA 22902

e-mail: hrpc@hrpub.com
www.hrpub.com